SK277 Human Biology
Science: Level 2

The Open University

Cells and Nutrition

This publication forms part of an Open University course SK277 *Human biology*. The complete list of texts which make up this course can be found at the back. Details of this and other Open University courses can be obtained from the Student Registration and Enquiry Service, The Open University, PO Box 197, Milton Keynes MK7 6BJ, United Kingdom: tel. +44 (0)870 333 4340, email general-enquiries@open.ac.uk

Alternatively, you may visit the Open University website at http://www.open.ac.uk where you can learn more about the wide range of courses and packs offered at all levels by The Open University.

To purchase a selection of Open University course materials visit www.ouw.co.uk, or contact Open University Worldwide, Walton Hall, Milton Keynes MK7 6AA, United Kingdom for a brochure (tel. +44 (0)1908 858793; fax +44 (0)1908 858787; email ouw-customer-services@open.ac.uk).

The Open University
Walton Hall, Milton Keynes
MK7 6AA

First published 2004. Second edition 2006.

Edited and designed by The Open University.

Typeset by The Open University.

Printed in the United Kingdom by Latimer Trend and Company Ltd, Plymouth.

The paper used in this publication is procured from forests independently certified to the level of Forest Stewardship Council (FSC) principles and criteria. Chain of custody certification allows the tracing of this paper back to specific forest-management units (see www.fsc.org).

ISBN 978 0 7492 1440 1

2.2

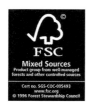

THE COURSE TEAM

Course Team Chair and Academic Editor

Heather McLannahan

Course Managers

Alastair Ewing

Colin Walker

Course Team Assistants

Catherine Eden

Rebecca Efthimiou

Course Team Authors

Patricia Ash

Pete Clifton

Paul Gabbott

Nicolette Habgood

Tim Halliday

Heather McLannahan

Kerry Murphy

Daniel Nettle

Payam Rezaie

Other Contributors

Vickie Arrowsmith

Leslie Baillie

Production and Presentation Manager

John Owen

Project Manager

Judith Pickering

Editors

Rebecca Graham

Gillian Riley

Bina Sharma

Margaret Swithenby

Design

Sarah Hofton

Jenny Nockles

Illustration

Steve Best

Pam Owen

CD-ROM Production

Phil Butcher

Will Rawes

External Course Assessor

Dinah Gould

Picture Researcher

Lydia Eaton

Indexer

Jane Henley

Course Website

Patrina Law

Louise Olney

SK277 *Human Biology* makes use of material originally produced for SK220 *Human Biology and Health* by the following individuals: Janet Bunker, Melanie Clements, Basiro Davey, Brian Goodwin, Linda Jones, Jeanne Katz, Heather McLannahan, Hilary MacQueen, Jill Saffrey, Moyra Sidell, Michael Stewart, Margaret Swithenby and Frederick Toates.

Cover image: © Alan Schein Photography/CORBIS

CONTENTS

CHAPTER 1

A BIOLOGICAL BASIS FOR HEALTH

Learning Outcomes

After completing this chapter, you should be able to:

1.1 Discuss the strengths and weaknesses of holistic and reductionist approaches to health and health care, using examples from biology, psychology and sociology.

1.2 Explain what is meant by biological determinism and the nature–nurture debate.

1.3 State the basic principles of Darwin's theory of biological evolution by natural selection.

1.4 Describe how epidemiological studies can be used to indicate possible causal factors in disease.

1.5 Explain the programming hypothesis and describe the proposed link between fetal environment and hypertension in later life.

1.1 Fact or fantasy?

Every day magazines and newspapers have articles, stories and advertisements that relate to our biology and health, but how can we judge their value? See, for example, the headlines presented in Figure 1.1 (overleaf).

Whilst there are clearly areas where even the 'experts' disagree the majority of us are better able to make up our own minds about the non-contentious issues when armed with some principles of human biology. So here we are, writing a course on human biology that we hope you will enjoy and also find useful and educational – especially when it comes to making personal health choices and reading the news.

Although the scientific study of the body has been the basis for modern medicine in the Western world for centuries, it has, in recent time, also led to an appreciation that there are other equally valid and interconnected ways of promoting health and combating disease. We will draw your attention to some of these connections as the course progresses but keep our focus on matters biological. **Biology** is the study of living organisms, their body structures and functions and their interrelationships. It is a diverse branch of science, with many subdisciplines of which the following will form the major portion of this course:

* **anatomy** – the study of the structures of the body;

* **physiology** – the study of the relationship between structure and function of body systems;

* **biochemistry** – the study of the chemical interactions that occur within the cells and fluids of the body;

* **behaviour** – the study of our activities and interactions.

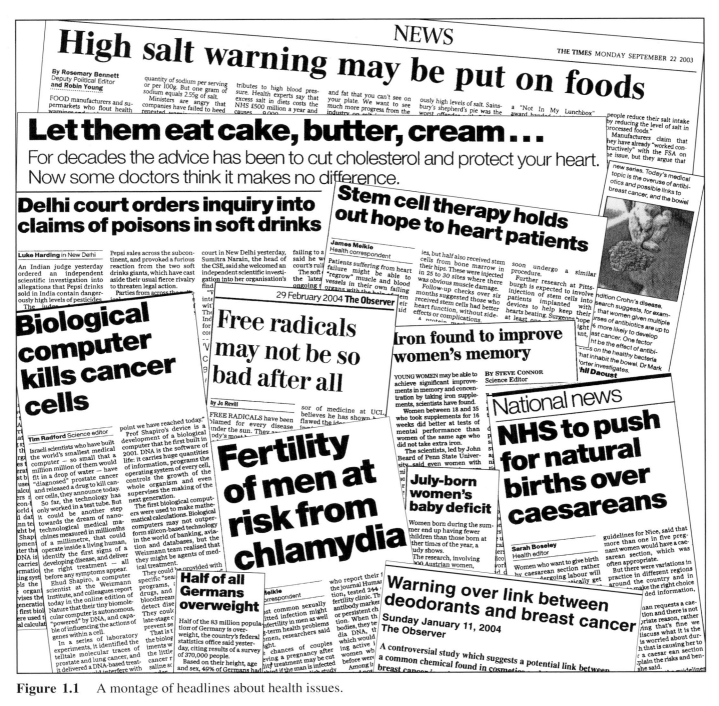

Figure 1.1   A montage of headlines about health issues.

Incidentally, there is a point we wish to make clear at the outset. Science is about the methods that are used to study, not about being 'right'. Too often we read that 'scientists tell us' or 'it is a scientific fact' only to discover that the 'fact' is hypothetical and currently purely speculative. The methods of scientific enquiry involve a cycle of activities that includes **hypothesis** formation but *starts* with an observation such as 'we breathe more rapidly and deeply (pant) after running'. This is followed by hypothesis construction, e.g. thinking of a reason why we pant after running, experimentation to test the hypothesis and incorporating data generation, data analysis, data interpretation and hypothesis reconstruction. Often this cycle of activities does result in establishing certainties; for example, in 1628 William Harvey showed how the heart pumped blood through the blood vessels of the body, with the **arteries** taking blood away from the heart and the **veins** returning it to the heart. But this immediately raised other questions: what keeps the heart beating, why does the heart have four chambers, what is the difference between venous and arterial blood; why is blood pumped round the body anyway?

● From general knowledge; why is blood circulated around the body?

● Blood is a transport medium. It carries nutrients and oxygen to all parts of the body and removes waste products.

The more we observe, the more questions bubble up. Good science should generate more questions than it answers. Indeed, as biology is the study of life and human biology the study of human life it is unsurprising that, in our vanity, much effort has been devoted to this branch of science. The reward is that in studying human biology we will be studying some of the great ideas of science. One of the most significant is Darwin's theory of natural selection (of which we will say more in Section 1.4.2). However, just as science is not about being 'right', nor is biology the means by which we can explain every aspect of human life.

1.2 Biological determinism and the nature–nurture debate

The belief that every aspect of human life – including attributes such as intelligence, personality and artistic talent – can ultimately be explained in terms of human biology is known as **biological determinism**. Advocates of this view claim that even though the organism expresses its characteristics in its behaviour and in the structure and activity of its cells, tissues and organs, the ultimate explanation for all its characteristics lies in the organism's *genes*. (There will be more about genes later on in the course, but for now even a vague idea is enough.) The argument, at its most extreme, states that genes direct a person's outward appearance, inner biological functioning, thoughts, feelings and behaviours as surely as if a puppet-master were pulling the strings.

In the 20th century, the *eugenics* movement gained supporters not only in Nazi Germany, but in many other parts of the world as well. For example, it was used to 'justify' the apartheid policy in South Africa and the so-called 'ethnic cleansing' in places such as Rwanda, as recently as 1994. Advocates of eugenics believed that there were genetic differences between races and between individuals, which gave inherent advantages and disadvantages in terms of intellect and other abilities. It was therefore morally right, they claimed, to prevent those with low inherent abilities from passing on their defective genes to future generations, and equally defensible for the master races to assume authority over the rest.

In the 21st century, we can hear the echoes of this philosophy in the claim that before long each of us will be carrying a 'smart card' imprinted with our personal genetic details. By implication, those found to have the 'healthiest' collection of genes could be awarded advantages in employment, insurance and possibly marriage or parenthood, which would be denied to, or at least made more expensive for, the rest. You will already have encountered examples of biological determinism in the media, as scientists announce the discovery of genes that they claim (variously) to be responsible for criminal behaviour, or homosexuality, or mathematical excellence, to name but a few. No doubt, there must be a genetic contribution to all of these attributes, but this is a far cry from asserting that genes alone are *responsible* for them.

Reducing human biology and health to the activity of human genes ignores the fact that the surrounding environment in which those genes operate has a profound influence on the ways in which their effects are manifested. For example, *susceptibility* to many complex diseases has a genetic component which acts together with environmental factors to promote disease.

- From your general knowledge, can you give any examples here?
- Looking at Figure 1.1 might have led you to suggest breast cancer. (There are, of course, many other valid suggestions that you might have made.)

In fact only around 5% of cases of breast cancer can be linked to the inheritance of particular genes. And whether the use of a deodorant increases the likelihood of developing cancer is a moot point. On a more positive note, *resistance* to many complex diseases has a genetic component which acts in concert with environmental factors to promote health. However, the focus on genes has frequently been at the expense of attempts to study the whole organism, undoubtedly in part because this is intrinsically difficult, but also because some biologists have argued that it was simply not a worthwhile enterprise. For example, Jim Watson – one of the scientists who worked out the structure of **DNA** (deoxyribonucleic acid, the complex chemical that contains genes within its structure) in the early 1950s – is reported to have said that 'everything else is merely social work'. When anyone takes such a narrow view whilst attempting an explanation of complex human phenomena such as 'health' we say they have taken a **reductionist** view. In effect, reductionist explanations reduce the possible interpretations of a complex phenomenon, such as a health issue like the spread of HIV/AIDS, to the domain covered by a single field of knowledge or belief. So, for example, to explain the spread of HIV/AIDS as an act of God is reductionist in the sense that a complete explanation is offered from within a single discipline – in this case, the religious one. All other apparent levels of explanation (genetic, physiological, social or psychological, for example) are either discarded as irrelevant or reinterpreted as subsidiary ramifications of the 'true' level. In the example we are pursuing here, if evidence for the spread of AIDS is found at (say) the biological level, then this can be reinterpreted as evidence that God controls all the biological manifestations of life itself. This example is worth emphasizing because the term reductionist sounds as though it means 'interprets complex phenomena in terms of their smallest possible constituents' and, indeed, it is often misused in this way; but in reality it means 'interprets complex phenomena in terms of a single discipline', which may be as vast as a divine creator.

- Is a belief in biological determinism reductionist?
- Yes.

- What would be the consequence of this single-minded attention to one discipline (the genetic)?

● Researchers would ignore all influences on complex phenomena falling outside that field of study and *interactions* between different influences would remain invisible.

To continue with our AIDS example, it would mean researchers belittling the possibility that there could be any worthwhile contribution from social and cultural studies in the fight to control the spread of the disease. This is important because attacks on the reputation of other disciplines can damage their ability to compete for research funds (and students).

For practical reasons we will frequently spend much time in consideration of just one scientific discipline, the biological. But it is our intention to ensure that we never leave a topic without reminding you that health issues must always take account of the contribution of other disciplines such as **psychology** (the study of our mental life) and **sociology** (the study of interactions between individuals within a society).

The interaction of genes and environment is at the heart of the so-called **nature–nurture debate**, an often badly formulated and thereby largely fruitless argument about 'how much' of a particular human characteristic is due to genetic inheritance (nature) and 'how much' to the influence of environmental factors (nurture). For example, how much of a person's intelligence is due to his or her genes and how much to nutrition, health and education during childhood? However, there are serious questions about the interaction of genes and the environment on growth and development, which have been investigated principally by studying identical twins who were separated at birth and brought up by different families: their genes are identical but they are raised in different environments. If they turn out to have different characteristics, then (in theory) these are likely to be due to differences in their environments.

There may be some useful purpose in determining the relative contributions of genes and environment to human growth and development, but the nature–nurture debate has been conducted mainly on ideological rather than practical grounds. The discovery of a number of diseases (e.g. cystic fibrosis) in which the inheritance of a *single* gene can profoundly damage a person's health, has lent support to arguments that *every* aspect of biological functioning will also turn out to be determined by genes, with little input from the environment. The opposing view has also been fiercely argued: that humans are products of their upbringing, social circumstances, education and access to resources, rather than the slaves of their genes.

Most biologists would now agree that nature and nurture interact. An often-quoted example demonstrates this point. Manipulation of the environment can prevent disease from developing in some individuals who have inherited a *lethal gene defect* – a faulty gene which causes fatal damage if its effects are not counteracted. Babies born with a faulty gene that prevents them from breaking down a common constituent of the diet (called phenylalanine), suffer brain damage as this substance builds up in the bloodstream (a condition known as **phenylketonuria**, or PKU for short). However, if the diet is controlled to exclude excess phenylalanine, then the damage cannot occur: changing the environment counteracts the effects of the gene.

● Is the explanation of PKU reductionist?

○ Yes, the explanation for the disease is given as being a consequence of a faulty gene, i.e. the explanation is a genetic one.

● In this instance would you say that taking a reductionist approach has been positive or negative?

○ This example of PKU shows a positive side to the reductionist approach. The very power of reductionist science is its ability to home in on the critical details of human biology, and to reveal the inner workings of the body – sometimes with amazing precision.

The fact that PKU can be successfully treated by dietary manipulation rests on knowledge of a single gene among around 30 000 others in human DNA, and its effect on a single molecule, phenylalanine, among the multitude of different kinds of molecule in the human body. This is reductionism in all its glory. By setting aside all distractions and focusing research on the smallest components of life, a wealth of information about human biology has been gathered – much of which has been put to good use. Reductionism in itself is not a bad thing. The problems that flow from it are the consequence of elevating biological science to the status of supreme truth. You may wish to read Case Report 1.1 now to gain an insight into how the condition of PKU is detected and treated.

Case Report 1.1 Phenylketonuria

Alice and David, both aged 28, have just had their first baby, a girl named Charlotte weighing 3.1 kg. Mother and baby are discharged home 48 hours later to the care of Jenny, the community midwife they met during the pregnancy. She checks that Alice is recovering from the birth, that breastfeeding is being established and that Charlotte is feeding well. When Charlotte is six days old Jenny explains that it is time to do the 'blood spot' test. David and Alice are aware of this test because Jenny left a leaflet on one of her earlier visits. The leaflet explains that it is a special screening test done on all new-born babies in the UK since 1969 to detect a range of diseases, including a metabolic disease called phenylketonuria (PKU). It involves pricking Charlotte's heel and allowing some blood to drop onto a special card, which is then sent to the screening laboratory.

Although concerned that the test might be painful for the baby, they give consent for the procedure and within a few minutes the sample of blood is taken and Charlotte settles back to sleep.

A few days later Alice and David receive a visit from Sally, the health visitor. They are distressed to be told that Charlotte has tested positive for phenylketonuria. Arrangements are in place for them to see the consultant paediatrician at the regional hospital the following day, when further tests are to be taken to confirm the diagnosis and to commence treatment. Sally spends time listening to their worries and answering their questions – she offers her support through the days ahead. When Alice expresses the thought that it must be something she did wrong during the pregnancy the couple are reminded that it is an inherited condition, though neither Alice nor David is aware of anyone in the family with PKU.

In response to their questions Sally tells them that because Charlotte has an enzyme missing in her body she is unable to use some protein foods properly, i.e. those containing phenylalanine. Normally any extra phenylalanine is turned into other proteins and used by the body. However, because this change is not working correctly there will be an excess of phenylalanine in the blood which will cause damage to the brain. In spite of this, with careful life-long dietary treatment they can expect Alice to lead a normal life.

At the hospital the next day the diagnosis is confirmed. The paediatrician explains that Charlotte will be closely monitored throughout her childhood by a multi-disciplinary team at a regional centre for PKU. The district general hospital and their GP will also monitor her development and give guidance and support on the management of her diet. The doctor outlines the treatment that Charlotte will receive and again reassures Alice and David that the outlook for children with PKU is good, but that they may consider having genetic counselling to discuss the risks of having another child with PKU. Because blood levels must be closely monitored, Alice and David will also receive instruction from a clinical nurse specialist on how to take samples of Charlotte's blood.

Meanwhile, to allow the levels of phenylalanine in her blood to fall Charlotte will immediately start a special formula milk low in phenylalanine. The paediatric dietician informs Alice that she cannot breastfeed until this has happened but that later she will be able to give a small amount of breast milk after the formula feed to make sure that Charlotte has adequate amounts of phenylalanine necessary to ensure her healthy growth and development. Additionally they will have support from Sally, their own health visitor, and will be put in touch with the National Society for PKU.

Summary of Section 1.2

1   Biological determinism is a belief that every characteristic of human life is genetically determined.

2   This particular reductionist view leads seamlessly into the nature–nurture debate by denying that environment is of significance in the development of human characteristics.

3   The example of PKU demonstrates that interactions between genes and environment determine the outcome of developmental processes.

1.3 Holism and reductionism in health care

As an alternative to the reductionist approach to a health issue we can attempt an interdisciplinary analysis. This could start with a review of what each of the relevant disciplines can contribute from within its field of expertise. In practice it is rarely (if ever) the case that any investigation or discussion of a health issue incorporates evidence from widely disparate disciplines. Attempts to do so are often termed **holistic** explanations, because they strive to keep the 'whole' in view, with all its many interacting possibilities.

The strengths and weaknesses of holistic and reductionist approaches to explanation can be illustrated by reference to health care.

1.3.1 Holistic approaches to health care

If we were able to give a fully integrated account of all the many and varied biological, psychological and sociological influences on human health, it could properly be termed holistic. However, keeping all the possible disciplines in view would be a hugely difficult task, requiring sophisticated and specialized knowledge of several fundamentally different areas of study. Not surprisingly, it is usual to find that a given health issue (like issues in many other fields) is investigated and discussed primarily within one discipline area – for example, the biological – with little more than lip service paid to the others. But even an acknowledgement that there are other valid ways of investigating the issue is to take a holistic *perspective*.

The words health and holism both have their roots in the concept of wholeness: health comes from the Anglo-Saxon word, and holism from the Greek word for whole. The two concepts were indivisible in medieval European culture, where sickness was understood to be a disorder of the whole person. The body was viewed as a vessel in which the four humours (blood, phlegm, yellow and black bile) intermingled under the influence of intrinsic qualities (hot, cold, wet and dry) and elements (earth, air, fire and water). Thus, in sickness, the whole person was in disharmony with inner and outer forces, and the return to health relied on restoring the balance between opposites. This understanding of the interdependence of body and mind remained a cornerstone in the philosophy and medicinal practices of the Eastern world. However, in the Western world, the rise of scientific medicine from the 18th century onwards drove out this view, replacing it with a model of health as the 'absence of disease'. The body was now viewed as a machine; in sickness a bit of the machinery had 'gone wrong' and just needed to be 'fixed' by the medical expert (doctor). Holistic concepts of health did not resurface in Western culture until about the 1950s, when the term 'biopsychosocial' began to be used in the context of the mental-health movement. Psychiatry was criticized for its focus on disease and reliance on drugs and other medical interventions, while ignoring the social, psychological, behavioural and cultural dimensions of the patient's experience and rehabilitation. In 1958, the World Health Organization (WHO) developed a holistic definition of health, as 'a state of complete physical, mental and social wellbeing' (WHO, 1958), and this definition continues to be enshrined in its Constitution.

The idea of considering the 'whole person' began to appear in nursing models of care far sooner than it did in medicine, with its emphasis on the 'doctor-centred' model of treating the disease rather than the patient. Nurses are now routinely educated to take account of the patient's psychological and social worlds, as well as their biological state. The concept of nurses aiding patients in caring for themselves (self-care) is playing an increasingly important part in how nurses see their role. Empowering the patient to self-care can be seen as liberating the patient from professional dominance. Alternatively, cynics claim that it is a way of running a health service more cheaply and with fewer trained staff, expecting patients and their friends and family to undertake most of the caring.

The holistic approach has been further strengthened in health care by the inclusion of some alternative or complementary therapies in the range of available treatment options. These therapies are 'alternative' to conventional medicine because they respond to the *person* who is seeking help to recover or maintain health, and engage that person as an active agent in the process. However, there are legitimate doubts about the extent to which these therapies are effective in treating or preventing illness and promoting well-being. This is at least partly because the reductionist scientific methods used to evaluate conventional therapies are not well suited to investigate the 'personalized' outcomes that alternative therapies claim to achieve. In recent years, collaborative research between alternative and conventional practitioners has been steadily increasing. A drawback for some users of alternative therapies is that taking personal responsibility for becoming ill is part and parcel of taking responsibility for getting well again. Holistic approaches to cancer treatment have been highly praised by many patients, but some have suffered the added distress of self-doubt and personal failure if they could not 'conquer' the disease.

A powerful advantage of holistic approaches to any complex phenomenon is that knowledge generated by one discipline can inform and enhance the investigations carried out in another field of study, and reveal the interactions between them. Curiously enough, one of the leading figures to promote such views – the English sociologist, David Armstrong – has also been a strong critic of the extent to which holism as a philosophy has begun to claim the moral high ground. Armstrong (1986) argues that it has become almost heretical to point out the limitations of holistic approaches to understanding human societies and social relations, particularly in the area of health and health care. Holistic approaches in any area of study have several weaknesses: for example, it can be hard to get anything done if all disciplines have to be included; potentially valuable single-discipline research can be underrated; and, since no-one has full command of all the knowledge and debates within every discipline, apparently holistic explanations often turn out to be superficial. If the holistic view of human health assumes the status of 'supreme truth' it is in danger of becoming reductionist!

1.3.2 Reductionist approaches to health care

Reductionism has been the dominant influence on Western medical thought for the past three centuries, and it has become fashionable for advocates of holistic health care to view this as malign. Certainly it has led to the person being 'reduced to' the disease, with no greater responsibility than to transport the symptoms to a doctor for diagnosis and treatment, and then to comply faithfully with instructions. People who delay seeking medical help tend to be chastized, as though the disease 'belongs' to the professionals. Patients have sometimes complained that they were expected to be passive recipients of medical care and accept that 'doctor knows best', but it is worth noting that confidence in orthodox medicine is justifiably widespread. If its successes have often been overplayed, they are nonetheless considerable.

● Give one example of a positive outcome of the reductionist approach.

◐ The diagnosis and treatment of PKU is a triumph of reductionism.

But the point of this chapter is not to rehearse the arguments about whether, and if so to what extent, Western medicine has been a success. The aim here is to reveal its reductionist credentials and point to the consequences. The basis of modern medicine is the scientific study of the human body, so disease has come to be understood as disordered functioning of specific parts of the body. The medical task is to identify the malfunction and put it right. The most disputed disease categories are those such as myalgic encephalomyelitis (ME, also known as post-viral fatigue syndrome) where no *consistent* physical damage or malfunction has been detected with the technology currently available, that reliably distinguishes these conditions from other related disorders. If the disease cannot be reduced to a precise description of this or that cellular or molecular derangement, then uncertainty about its legitimacy cannot be banished. This philosophy has led to considerable frustration and misery for people who feel ill but cannot 'prove' their illness exists, according to the criteria set by the reductionist nature of medical science.

Reductionism in medicine has also meant that the outcomes of orthodox medical interventions are categorized as either 'central' effects or 'side' effects – a view that tends to undervalue the importance of side-effects for *patients* as long as the central effect is to counteract the *disease*. For example, the surgical treatment of breast cancer by mastectomy was conducted for many years without much consideration given to its psychological side-effects on women. However, the power of reductionist science has enabled a huge range of useful drugs, vaccines and surgical interventions to be developed, and there is little serious argument that they should be abandoned in favour of alternative therapies that claim to be holistic. The movement in modern health care seems to be towards a greater partnership between reductionist and holistic approaches, as outlined in the next section.

1.3.3 Developing a fruitful dialogue

We should, by now, have dispelled the false notion that holism is 'good' and reductionism is 'bad' by noting the strengths and weaknesses of each approach. It is our intention in this book – and in the course as a whole – to foster a dialogue between these two approaches, while using each of them to their best advantage. One of our aims is to encourage you to travel more easily between these often falsely opposed poles.

The discussion of holism in health care in late 20th-century industrialized countries can be seen as a rediscovery of the *variety* of ways of looking at, and caring for, health. In place of the medical model, a collaborative multidisciplinary team approach is increasingly being advocated, in which the patient is a key team member along with a range of professionals. This is exemplified by the 'Expert Patient' programme (Department of Health, 2001). However, the coordination and resources necessary to bring all these agencies together and the educational task in teaching them to speak a common language presents a huge challenge. But by studying human health as a multidimensional and dynamic phenomenon, it is hoped that new understanding will emerge and new methods of tackling health problems will be developed. It is our aim in this course to foster that development.

Summary of Section 1.3

1   Both reductionist and holistic approaches to health care have strengths and weaknesses.

2   In this course we intend to encourage integration between these two approaches.

1.4 Evolution and human health

It may seem as though we are now heading off into a completely new topic, but there are two reasons for bringing evolution into the discussion at this point. First, it is an area of undisputed importance for human health, which has nonetheless provoked bitter controversy between holistic and reductionist interpretations of evolution that continue to the present day. So in one sense it is an instructive 'case study' of what we have been discussing in previous sections. Second, it is also essential for you to understand something of the processes of evolution, so it is useful to get an overview of evolutionary change before you meet these terms again.

1.4.1 Biological and cultural evolution

We start by making a distinction between *biological evolution* and *cultural evolution*, because these two processes differ in what they transmit to future generations and in the mechanisms they use. **Biological evolution** involves the transmission of genes, the basic units of inheritance, which are passed on from parents to offspring in their eggs and sperm (a process which is discussed further later in this course). **Cultural evolution** involves the handing down of social customs and values, and knowledge passed on from teacher to pupil; it is also transmitted in artefacts such as books, technologies of many kinds, and works of art and architecture.

There is a vast difference in terms of time-scales. From the moment that the earliest life forms appeared on Earth perhaps 3500–4000 million years ago there have been gradual changes to the structures and functions of living things. By contrast the gradual changes to the customs, beliefs, values, knowledge and actions of human societies have only been occurring for about the last two million years or so. In both cases, what is passed down to one generation differs in some respects from the inheritance of previous generations, so the forms and structures of biology and culture both 'evolve' – they change over time. Moreover, they *interact* and this has great importance for human health.

Fossil evidence tells us that the organisms we refer to as modern humans emerged around 200 000 years ago, and that aspects of human culture have been influencing human biology, and vice versa, ever since. For example, cultural changes in diet and food preparation have had an impact on human biology in terms of the structure of our digestive tracts, bones and teeth. The anatomical features required to grind down raw foods have gradually changed, and the cultural 'breakthrough' of harnessing fire for cooking enabled humans to exploit a huge new range of foodstuffs. As new foods and hence new **habitats** (places to live) became accessible, communities of humans spread into them, and new cultures evolved. Biological changes occur much more slowly than cultural change: the human appendix may be one vestige of a portion of the digestive tract that was useful in the very distant past, but which now has no known digestive function and may gradually disappear in the far distant future.

Despite their different time-scales, it is important to recognize that the influences between human biology and human culture are two-way: they interpenetrate (i.e. they reciprocally interact with each other). This process is demonstrated if we consider the *environment* in which both biological and cultural evolution take place.

● What does the term 'environment' mean to you?

◉ In everyday language, the environment is often taken to mean the physical world around us – land masses, rivers, mountains, etc. and their vegetation, together with the built environment of cities and roads. A wider definition includes the climate and weather, the quality and availability of food, water and air, and the amounts of natural and industrial radiation.

Biologists add to this all the other organisms sharing the same habitat, including microscopic ones such as bacteria. Psychologists would use the term to include any feature of the external world that influences human behaviours or mental states. Social scientists and historians would include all the aspects of culture and technology that characterize human societies. (Indeed your definition of environment might well have included financial, political or other aspects of our intellectual life.)

In the discussion that follows, we are using 'environment' in this all-inclusive sense, which encompasses the physical, biological, psychological and social worlds in continuous interaction.

1.4.2 Evolution and natural selection

If biological evolution is the history of biological change, what are the forces that prompt change to occur? This is an area of considerable agreement between biologists – even those who sit in opposing camps when it comes to discussing the relative contributions of genes (nature) and environment (nurture) to the outcome.

The theory of biological evolution by natural selection is associated with the British naturalist Charles Darwin (1809–1882), who noted the range of *variation* in appearance and behaviour even among the members of a single **species** – that is, a population of similar organisms that usually interbreed in their natural habitat and produce fertile offspring. This variation is extremely important because it provides the potential for the species to survive environmental change. If the conditions in a certain environment gradually alter – for example, because the average temperature rises, or the environment becomes overcrowded – some members of the species will find it easier to survive than others, because tiny differences in their body structure, or function, or behaviour, give them a small advantage. For example, if the average temperature rises, then individuals who are better able to lose excess heat (perhaps because they have less body hair, or produce more sweat) will be at a slight advantage.

The characteristics of body structure, or function, or behaviour, which give some members of a species a survival advantage, are termed **adaptive characteristics**. If the advantage is sufficiently great, then the proportion of better-adapted individuals who survive long enough to reproduce and leave surviving offspring will exceed the proportion of less well-adapted survivors. This is the basis of natural selection, the driving force of evolution as described by Darwin. The theory relies on the fact that a population produces more offspring than can survive to parent the next generation, because the resources available in terms of food, shelter and so on are insufficient for all. In the competition for resources, a natural process of 'selection' occurs in that individuals with the most adaptive characteristics in the context of *that* environment at *that* time are the most likely to survive and reproduce. This principle is often translated as 'survival of the fittest' – a phrase that needs to be used with care, because it has the power to mislead in two ways.

First, we have to distinguish between the meaning of 'fittest' in everyday language and its meaning in evolutionary biology. Depending on the environmental conditions, the 'fittest' members of a species could be the slowest, sleepiest and most obese – if these characteristics give them a survival advantage over the rest. Second, the characteristics that denote the 'fittest' at any given time and place are not 'the best' characteristics in any absolute sense.

● Will the same individuals still be the fittest members of a species if the environmental conditions change, even by a little?

○ No; the accolade of 'fittest' will pass to other individuals with slightly different characteristics, who now find themselves better able to survive and reproduce in the new conditions than they were before.

To a biologist, then, **fitness** means *lifetime reproductive success* (i.e. the total number of surviving offspring) relative to the number produced by other members of the same species. But why is there this emphasis on reproductive success? A characteristic is only considered to be adaptive in an evolutionary sense if it can be passed on from parent to offspring. In other words the character must be **heritable**, and biological heritability is based on inheriting genes from your parents. Thus, the survival advantage conferred on the parent by an adaptive characteristic is also enjoyed by the offspring. Over many generations, if the characteristic continues to give an advantage, then the proportion of individuals in the species who share that characteristic can be expected to increase.

● Can you explain why?

○ More offspring of the better-adapted individuals will survive to reproduce in their turn; more of *their* offspring will survive to reproduce, and so on. At the same time, fewer offspring of the less well-adapted individuals will survive, because they lose out in the competition for resources. Consequently, the proportion of individuals in the species who share the adaptive characteristic rises.

1.4.3 Variation and change

If environments stayed the same, the members of a species would (in theory) become more and more adapted to survive and reproduce successfully in that environment from one generation to the next. But in reality, *environments never stay the same*. The natural world is in a continual state of change, so evolution by natural selection cannot produce 'perfection'. It is a common misconception to think of evolution as a process of 'onward and upward', when a better analogy might refer to a process of 'continually moving the goalposts'! The variation within a species is its strength: the species *as a whole* has a chance of surviving continual environmental change if its members have sufficient variation between individuals, such that some of them will survive when conditions change.

One of the beneficial outcomes of understanding evolutionary theory in this way is that it enables us to view human variation in a rather different light. Humans display immense variation – each face, each set of fingerprints is unique for over six billion individuals, and that's just counting the ones alive today. The ability to colonize almost every habitat on Earth, from the deserts to the ice-caps and everything in between, is a testament to human evolution by natural selection which has resulted in so many variations on a basic theme. This variability is our protection against extinction. Species such as the dodo and the dinosaurs paid the ultimate price when the environment changed around them: the variations between individuals were insufficiently great and none could survive and reproduce in the new conditions. So, from a biological standpoint alone, the intolerance that human societies often display towards individuals who look different and behave differently from the norm is illogical.

1.4.4 Nature and nurture revisited

This is the point at which we head into more troubled waters and revisit the earlier debates about nature and nurture in the context of evolution. Just as there has been argument about the *sufficiency* of genes to explain everything about the structure and function of the individuals we see around us today, the role of genes in the vast timescale of biological evolution is also open to debate.

All biologists agree that characteristics are passed on from one generation to the next in the form of genes, donated from parents to offspring in sexually reproducing species such as ourselves, in the eggs and sperm. Organisms survive or die out in a given environment because variations between individuals confer advantages on those with the best-adapted characteristics. Since many of these variations are a consequence of variations in the genes each individual has inherited, so natural selection can be said to be 'selecting' organisms with the best-adapted genes in that environmental context. The problem lies in deciding whether anything *in addition to* genetic inheritance should also be taken into account when considering evolutionary change.

There is at one extreme, a gene-centred theory of evolution popularized by the biologist Richard Dawkins in his book *The Selfish Gene* (1976), which views organisms as nothing more than vehicles for ensuring the survival of genes. In this highly reductionist account, all the characteristics of an organism (behavioural, psychological and physical) can be traced to the activity of its genes. This theory has been enormously influential in popular culture as a result of its promotion in documentaries, best-selling books and newspaper articles. It leads to a view of the body as a collection of interacting and more-or-less independent parts – analogous to a construction model kit in which parts can be removed, added or modified independently of each other without fundamentally changing the nature of the model itself. In terms of evolutionary change, if a 'part' is useful to the survival of the organism as a whole, then this theory predicts it will be found increasingly in future generations; if not, then it will gradually fade out of the species. Since the 'parts' themselves are programmed to have certain characteristics by the organism's genes, then it can be said that the individual genes – rather than the whole organism – are subject to natural selection.

Critics of this view of evolution argue that it presents organisms as opportunistic 'survival machines', with no other function than to pass on their genes to as many offspring as possible. In sharp contrast, the holistic view of evolutionary change sees organisms as more than the 'sum of their parts'; this theory argues that evolution has produced organisms which are complex integrated wholes. To return to the construction kit analogy, parts within the model are not independently variable and dispensable; parts could not change independently of changes to the model as a whole. This approach to an understanding of evolution asserts, just as Darwin did, that whole organisms are subject to natural selection.

Supporters of this holistic view of evolutionary change offer three arguments in making their case. First, humans and other organisms don't have perfectly adapted bodies so – despite natural selection – there are some genes preserved in the species which confer less-than-optimum characteristics (for example, the genes that influence the development of the appendix in humans). According to the gene-centred theory of evolutionary change, these genes ought to 'die out', unless you construct an argument that says 'well, there must be other genes that ensure the preservation of these less-than-optimum genes'. The logic then begins to get circular! Health depends upon a combination of heredity and habit, of nature and nurture. We don't have perfect bodies – over time there have been compromises. After all, our ancestors had tails and we have lost them, except for a remnant that is quite prominent in the early human embryo (Figure 1.2). All we can say is that some organs appear to be more difficult to modify or eliminate than others, but this is not an explanation. Rather, it points to an interesting problem and to the second argument that counters the gene-centred theory of evolution.

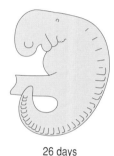

26 days

Figure 1.2   The external form of the human embryo at 26 days showing the 'tail' (actual size ×16).

The second argument is that it appears that there may be constraints on the construction of body structures. Consider this example. In every four-limbed animal that exists or (on fossil evidence) has ever existed, the limb starts at the shoulder or pelvis with a single long bone, which then makes a joint with two bones (elbow or knee), and these then articulate with a complex of bones ending in a number of digits. This structure is known as the *tetrapod limb*. No-one disputes that variations on this theme (e.g. compare the limbs of a gazelle, a frog and a human) are adaptations to life in different environments, but no matter how useful it might be to have a different *basic* limb structure, evolutionary processes have not produced an alternative to the tetrapod limb in millions of years. You might think that in some species it would be more useful to have two bones to start with – for example, birds need a strong, light, flat structure for the wing, and two struts together can be lighter and stronger than one. However, since no such structure has emerged, it could be argued that there may be *intrinsic* constraints on how the body is constructed – no matter which genes you inherit. Constraints such as this may account for many aspects of our body structures which are certainly not optimal, but work well enough. At the level of the individual, genes impose fundamental biological limits on each individual's capacity to grow and develop, and to respond to disturbances that affect health. This is most obvious when a person inherits genes with altered structures that interfere with normal biological functioning, but it is equally true (though often forgotten) that the state of 'bounding health' also has inherited and relatively stable biological components.

Third, the gene-centred theory ignores the *interpenetration* of organism and environment. Since all species modify their environments, they transmit not only their genes but an altered environment to successive generations as a result of their behaviour. Humans do this more than any other species: we are undeniably transmitting an altered environment to our progeny which is favourable to their survival in some respects and unfavourable in others. The open question is the extent to which the environment we inherit is acting on our genes, at the same time as our genes are acting on the environment!

To conclude, there is a consensus in biology that genes set limits to the *range* of behaviour, body structures and functions that any individual can express, while the environment or culture adds a further component of specificity in determining *which* of the possibilities an individual actually expresses. Health depends on a combination of genetic inheritance and environmental factors, of nature and nurture. To attempt to disentangle and measure their *relative* influence is fraught with difficulty. However, the reductionist tradition in biology sees the task as a useful pursuit of knowledge, while the holistic tradition decries it as an attempt to rip apart an indivisible whole.

We, like all the other species on our planet, are involved in a continuously creative process that results from, and depends upon, diversity and the ability to negotiate change – of individuals, species, environments and cultures. Health can then be seen as a creative response to whatever circumstances are encountered, so it involves a different strategy for each person. Health is an expression of this integrated whole, which involves living with compromises and imperfections.

Summary of Section 1.4

1   An understanding of the Darwinian theory of evolution by natural selection enables us to appreciate how changes can occur within human populations over long periods of time.

2   Whilst genes set constraints on the characteristics that can be expressed, the environment determines what actually happens.

1.5 The biological foundations of health

Many environmental factors that affect our biology and health appear to be of our own, very personal making. There has recently been a strong emphasis on the importance of lifestyle in connection with health. In particular, a poor diet, lack of exercise and smoking have been strongly linked to one of the primary causes of death in the affluent industrialized nations, namely **cardiovascular disease** (diseases of the heart and blood vessels). The most familiar symptom is high blood pressure (**hypertension**), which is associated with strokes and heart attacks. In making these observations we are noting correlations.

●   Do you think that noting a correlation between lack of exercise and heart disease *proves* that lack of exercise causes heart disease?

● No. A correlation does not prove causality.

When two events are correlated it may be that a third event has caused both of them to occur. As an example, suppose that you notice that the chimes of two nearby church clocks always strike within a few seconds of each other. The clock that always strikes first could be causing the second to strike, or they could be working independently and slightly out of phase in response to some other (unobserved) factor or cue. It is possible to determine which hypothesis is correct by means of an experiment; in this case, one would stop the first clock and see whether the second still struck at the expected time.

However, sometimes it is not possible to make such a direct experimental intervention and we may have to be satisfied with more indirect evidence. In some instances this may initially rest on a single observation. Where the observation is of just a single individual, it is called an anecdote, or **case report**, depending on who does the observing and where they make their observation known. So if I observe that my friend has become very depressed since her husband left her and has lost a considerable amount of weight, or if a newspaper or magazine reports similarly a weight loss in a film star who has suffered a broken relationship, then this story, however true, is an anecdote. A similar story of events leading up to the onset of a medical condition such as anorexia (loss of appetite followed by loss of weight) reported by a trained scientist (e.g. a medical doctor, a physiologist or a psychologist), written about in medical journals or reported to medical conferences is a case report. The distinction between the case report and the anecdote rests partly on the experience and the authority of the observer, i.e. professional versus lay person.

Case reports may be informative, they are invariably interesting, and they may provide the basis of a theory, but they do not provide good evidence from which to generalize about the population. Rather more than one observation is needed to make general statements and to substantiate a theory – case reports need corroboration. One potential method of corroborating a case report may be to undertake an epidemiological study. **Epidemiology** involves a study in which relationships are sought between particular factors suspected of influencing contraction of disease and measures of health in communities and populations. This can take different forms, among which are *geographical studies* in which the incidences of particular diseases in different parts of the country are compared and related to other observations. For example, a Medical Research Council Environmental Epidemiology Unit at Southampton University noticed a paradox: the connection between lifestyle and health predicts that increasing affluence, resulting in heavier eating and less exercise, should increase the risk of cardiovascular disease. However, in the UK these diseases are commoner among poorer people. For instance, it is known that regions of the country that currently show high mortality from heart disease used to have high infant mortality, which is associated with poverty through inadequate nutrition, poor housing, stressful living and similar influences. The Southampton Group wondered if factors that adversely affect infant health might also cause disease in later life; that is, conditions to which the developing embryo in the womb and the early infant are exposed might have significant influences on health in the adult. To examine this possibility, the Group set up studies of individuals by using data more than 40 years old that gave relevant information about early development in the womb and early infancy in a group of people who had lived all their lives in a certain region. This kind of study is a **longitudinal study**. In longitudinal studies data on individuals are examined at different stages of life to see what factors may be influencing health over the life cycle. We will now consider this work.

1.5.1 Epidemiology: a longitudinal study

This study depended upon finding accurate records on individuals that gave relevant information about the conditions they experienced as developing embryos during pregnancy and as infants, and gathering data on the health of these individuals much later in their lives. Such data are not easy to come by, and you might think that the Southampton Group would have to set up a study with a cohort of pregnant women and wait for 40–50 years to examine the health of the individuals, then identifying whatever relationships emerged between early life and later health. However, this is hardly a practicable procedure since members of the group, and possibly the Medical Research Council itself, would not necessarily survive to complete the experiment.

- ● Can you think of a more scientific reason why setting up such a study now, to harvest data 50 years hence, is not a good procedure?

- ● Because scientific understanding changes so rapidly, the questions being asked now are likely to be seen as obsolete or irrelevant in 50 years time, and the kinds of information which would be sought then will include many items not originally recorded.

- ● In this context, is there an example within your own experience of a significant shift in attitude towards health or health therapies that has happened in the past 10 years or so, and that might affect the type of questions asked about health and lifestyle today?

- ● You may have noticed changes in lifestyle reflected by more joggers on the road, smoke-free zones in workplaces, restaurants, etc.; you may have encountered more people discussing and using complementary therapies such as homeopathy, aromatherapy, reflexology, acupuncture and spiritual healing, and these or others being offered at your local clinic.

The procedure followed by the Southampton Group was to search throughout the country for old maternity and infant welfare records that would provide relevant data on individuals now in their 40s or older. One such set of records was found at the Sharoe Green Hospital in Preston, Lancashire (Barker et al., 1990). Detailed information was available on infants born during the period 1935–43, including the baby's birth weight, placental weight, length from crown to heel, and head circumference. Those individuals who still lived in Lancashire in 1989, when the study was conducted (and so were in the age range 46–54), were traced and invited to participate in the investigation. This involved a visit by an investigator who recorded the following data: height, weight, blood pressure and pulse rate (with participants sitting down). The individuals were asked about their medical history, current medication, smoking habits, alcohol consumption and family history of cardiovascular disease. The father's occupation was used to define social class at birth, and current social class was derived from the participant's or her husband's occupation. After the interview blood pressure was measured again (participant seated throughout the interview) and the average of the two readings was used, to provide a more reliable measurement.

● Can you think of any other reason why the investigators wanted the blood pressure measurements to be taken twice?

◐ Sometimes people can be anxious at the start of an interview and this can lead to increased blood pressure. By the end of the interview they might be more relaxed and thus have a lower blood pressure reading.

The investigator had not seen the birth data recorded for the participants. This is known as working 'blind', often expressed as 'blind testing' or 'blind trials' in experiments. This technique is designed to avoid unconscious observer bias.

Blood pressure measurements usually include two values: a higher pressure recorded just after the heart has contracted (**systolic pressure**) and a lower value recorded while the heart is relaxed and filling with blood (**diastolic pressure**). The pressure is registered as the height in millimetres (mm) of a column of mercury (Hg) which the pressure supports (1 millimetre = 0.001 metres). (Chapter 2 of Book 3 gives more detail of the cardiovascular system.) Weight was recorded in pounds. Table 1.1 presents some results of the analysis. On the left is the baby's birth weight, recorded as less than 5.5 lb (< 5.5), between 5.5 and 6.5 lb (5.5–6.5), between 6.5 and 7.5 lb (6.5–7.5) and greater than 7.5 lb (> 7.5). Placental weight appears along the top, divided into groups of less than 1.0 lb (< 1), between 1.0 and 1.25 lb (1.0–1.25), and so on.

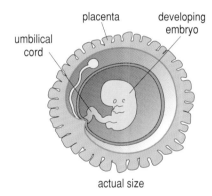

Figure 1.3   The developing embryo at 48 days showing the placenta and umbilical cord.

● The placenta is known colloquially as the 'after-birth'; from your general knowledge state its function.

◐ The placenta is the organ where the blood supplies of mother and developing embryo are closely juxtaposed (Figure 1.3). Through the placenta the embryo is supplied with nutrients and oxygen and waste products are removed.

Systolic pressure is entered as the average for the individuals falling into different categories, the numbers of individuals in the category being recorded in parentheses beside the average systolic pressure. For example, 77 individuals had birth weights between 6.5 and 7.5 lbs, and placental weights between 1.0 and 1.25 lb, and their average systolic pressure was 148 mmHg. The average systolic pressure for all individuals within a birth weight range, irrespective of placental weight, is presented in the *column* headed 'all', with the number of individuals in the range shown in parentheses. The *row* marked 'all' shows the other average: the average systolic pressure for all individuals whose placental weight falls into a certain range, irrespective of birth weight. The lower part of the table gives the diastolic pressures for the same groups as the upper part.

Table 1.1 Average systolic and diastolic blood pressures of men and women aged 46–54, according to placental weight and birth weight. Numbers of individuals in the category are shown in parentheses.

Birth weight/lb	Placental weight/lb				
	< 1.0	1.0–1.25	1.25–1.5	> 1.5	All
	Systolic pressure/mmHg				
< 5.5	152 (26)	154 (13)	153 (5)	206 (1)	154 (45)
5.5–6.5	147 (16)	151 (54)	150 (28)	166 (8)	151 (106)
6.5–7.5	144 (20)	148 (77)	145 (45)	160 (27)	149 (169)
> 7.5	133 (6)	148 (27)	147 (42)	154 (54)	149 (129)
All	147 (68)	149 (171)	147 (120)	157 (90)	150 (449)
	Diastolic pressure/mmHg				
< 5.5	84	87	87	97	86
5.5–6.5	84	88	85	93	87
6.5–7.5	84	84	84	90	85
> 7.5	78	85	85	88	86
All	84	86	85	89	86

A very rough indication of average systolic pressure for people older than 40 is given by the formula 100 + age.

● What range of systolic pressures would be expected for the sample of individuals in this investigation, using the above formula?

◗ Since the individuals were in the age range 46–54, the average systolic pressures would be expected to fall in the range 146–154 mmHg.

● Do the figures in Table 1.1 conform to this expectation?

◗ The overall average for the whole group is 150 mmHg, which is right in the middle of the expected range. The subgroups averaged for each of the four birth weight categories are in the range 149–154 mmHg, which is also within the expected range of 146–154 mmHg. But there are also groups whose average values fall outside the expected range, either below (133, 144 mmHg) or above (160, 166, 206 mmHg).

Using the table, answer the following questions.

● What is the relationship between birth weight and systolic pressure for individuals with placental weights of less than 1 lb?

◗ As birth weight increases, systolic pressure decreases. This is known as an **inverse relationship**.

● Is this inverse relationship followed consistently in each of the columns corresponding to different ranges of placental weight?

● No. In the third column (placental weight between 1.25 and 1.5 lb), the lowest systolic pressure (145 mmHg) is for individuals with birth weights between 6.5 and 7.5 lb, while in those with weights greater than 7.5 lb, it rises to 147 mmHg. However, the overall trend in the data is the same.

● Is the same trend shown in diastolic pressures?

● The trend is there, but it is very much weaker.

● What is the relationship between placental weight and systolic pressure for individuals with birth weights greater than 7.5 lb?

● There is a tendency for systolic pressure to increase as placental weight increases.

● Is the same tendency shown in the other rows?

● Yes.

The trends that occur in the data have to be checked for reliability by statistical methods, which allow one to determine the probability that such trends could appear just by chance, for the number of individuals measured. Clearly the more individuals, the more reliable is any trend revealed by the analysis. The numbers involved in this study allow for confidence in the conclusion that large placental weight and low body weight at birth are both correlated with higher blood pressure in later life. The Southampton Group analysed these data in many different ways to examine the relationships within them. In particular, they analysed the connection with hypertension, defined as a systolic pressure of greater than 160 mmHg. The strongest indicator of risk is given by the combination of placental weight and birth weight: highest blood pressures and risk of hypertension were among people who had been small babies with large placentas.

● What relationship would you expect to find between the weights of the adults in the Preston study and their blood pressures, and also between alcohol consumption and blood pressure, based on a connection between lifestyle and health?

● Both higher weight and higher alcohol consumption would be expected to correlate with higher blood pressure, and they did.

This finding is in agreement with the results of many other studies on the relationship between lifestyle and blood pressure. However, the relation of placental weight and birth weight to blood pressure was stronger, and it was independent of current body weight and alcohol consumption. That is to say, a large baby with a small placenta will tend to result in an adult with lower blood pressure, irrespective of lifestyle (as measured by the two indicators of alcohol consumption and weight), and conversely for a small baby with a large placenta. The two measurements taken at birth – weight of baby and weight of placenta – provide better predictors of blood pressure and hypertension than do lifestyle measures of the adult.

The study just described produced unexpected results and has provoked considerable comment and criticism. A single piece of work of this type could hardly stand on its own as a significant contribution to understanding the causes of cardiovascular disease. It has to be combined with many other studies that point in the same direction before one can be confident about the relationships that are indicated. The Southampton Group has produced an impressive amount of evidence from different analyses – both its own and those of other groups – supporting their hypothesis that there is a significant connection between the environment experienced by the developing embryo and the young infant, and later health (Barker, 1992). Lifestyle certainly influences health, but not as much as the earliest conditions of the developing individual. Measures of health used in these studies included not just blood pressure but susceptibility to respiratory infection, capacity to use glucose efficiently (related to diabetes), concentrations of fibrinogen in the blood (related to blood clot formation), among others. These all support the basic hypothesis about early environment and later disease.

However, there are many in the community of epidemiologists who are critical of the conclusions of the Southampton Group, and for good scientific reasons. They point to extensive studies carried out in other countries that failed to establish any connection between birth weight and blood pressure in late adolescence, for example, or which indicated the *opposite* relationship to the results obtained by the Southampton Group. Such disagreements are an intrinsic part of the scientific dialogue (as we pointed out at the start of this chapter) and have their origins in many different aspects of the research. Different studies are carried out in different ways, using different numbers of individuals, of different ages and in different countries. These introduce sources of variation that need to be investigated by yet more research to identify the factors responsible for the differences.

Another criticism is that the data might be explained by genetic mechanisms that determine both the blood pressure of the child *and* growth of the placenta.

●   If this were true, what kind of relationship would there be between blood pressure and placental weight?

●   The relationship would be a correlation, with both factors linked to the genetic mechanism. The genetic mechanism would be the causal factor.

It is known that mothers' blood pressures are related to those of their children. So it is possible that placental weight is linked to adult blood pressure by a genetic mechanism that somehow determines both the blood pressure of the child and the growth of the placenta. To test this, the Southampton Group used data from a study by another investigator on 5161 women undergoing a first pregnancy in Oxford during 1987–8 (Barker et al., 1990). This study used the blood pressures recorded at their first antenatal clinic attendance and examined relationships with birth weight of their babies, and placental weight. No correlations were found, so these results fail to support the hypothesis of a genetic link that could explain the observed connections.

There is no doubt that genes have a role to play in every aspect of an individual's development. However, this does not mean that now the Human Genome Project has mapped all the genes of the human body we understand how the human body is made and how defective genes cause genetic disease. This is partly because we don't yet know the roles of many of the mapped genes but also because genes are only one set of contributory factors to the intricate process that is the life experience of an individual. The tangled web that links together gene activity, environmental influence and personal lifestyle is complex and subtle, and the different strands contribute in different ways at different times and circumstances. Each one has to be examined to find the dominant influences in particular contexts.

1.5.2 The programming hypothesis

The evidence that conditions experienced by the developing embryo in the womb can affect the health of the individual in later life has given rise to a hypothesis about how this may come about, called the **programming hypothesis**. It is known from studies on animals that undernourishment of pregnant rats results in stunted growth of the offspring, and that this cannot be reversed by feeding an optimum diet after birth. Even short-term exposure of embryos or new-born animals to abnormal conditions can irreversibly affect the condition of the individual later on. For instance, a female rat injected with a small amount of testosterone during the first four days of life will develop perfectly normally until puberty. But then the animal fails to ovulate or to show normal female sexual behaviour. Some irreversible change has evidently occurred to the processes that are involved in the development of female reproductive activity. However, this happens only if the injection is given during the first four days following birth; after this period it has no effect. For rats, then, the first four days of life is the *sensitive period* for sexual maturation.

The different organs and systems of the human body develop in the embryo at different times, and they each have their sensitive periods during which they are particularly prone to external influences. We will return to this briefly in the final book of this course. The Southampton Group has used this knowledge to propose a programming hypothesis that could explain their observations. Because an embryo has sensitive periods in its development, environmental influences can affect its pathway of development and push the embryo into a permanently altered condition which has consequences for the future health of the individual. It can be said to have been reprogrammed relative to the developmental path of an embryo that did not experience the stressful environmental conditions. Thus we have the programming hypothesis. In relation to the results of the Preston study just described (Table 1.1) it leads to the question: what influences on the embryo could induce a large placental-to-birth weight ratio and at the same time result in a baby that is prone to the development of hypertension more than 40 years later?

1.5.3 Seeing life as a whole

It is known from studies on animals that if there is a reduced amount of nutrients or oxygen (a consequence of smoking) in the mother's blood, so that the embryo experiences malnutrition or **hypoxia** (reduced oxygen), then there is a redistribution of the blood from the embryonic heart such that proportionately more goes to the brain than to the body. This redistribution is a regulatory process that protects the brain from adverse conditions and is at the expense of the body (though the developing brain is relatively insensitive to changes of oxygen level until late in the pregnancy). The result is that the young have disproportionately large heads relative to the size of their bodies, though both tend to be smaller than in new-born animals that have experienced normal nutrient and oxygen supplies. It is also known that placentas tend to grow larger if the availability of oxygen or nutrients to the embryo is reduced. For example, mothers who are **anaemic** (deficient in **haemoglobin**, the oxygen-carrying protein in the blood) have a tendency to develop larger placentas. The same occurs with malnutrition: if the mother is undernourished, the placenta will tend to grow larger in an attempt, so to speak, to get more of the available nourishment for the embryo, though, in general, the embryo will still experience some malnutrition and so be on the small side. In both instances, of hypoxia and malnutrition, the growth and development of the head is favoured over the body.

● What prediction could be made about the ratio of head to body size in babies with large placentas and small birth weights?

● Because a large placental to birth weight ratio might result from either hypoxia or malnutrition (or both) in the mother, the regulatory mechanism that favours growth of the brain over that of the body under these circumstances would result in babies with small bodies relative to head size.

Since the Preston study (Section 1.5.1) included measurements of heel to crown length and head circumference of the new-born babies, this prediction could be checked. It was found that greater placental weight at any birth weight of the baby is associated with a decreased ratio of length to head circumference. So this is consistent with the possibility that a significant factor in the development of hypertension in adults is the experience of malnutrition and/or hypoxia by the embryo. The placenta would then overgrow in an attempt to compensate for these adverse conditions, but the result is likely to be babies with small bodies relative to head size. We now need to find a reason why such babies are at risk of developing hypertension as adults.

A possible link proposed by the Southampton Group involves the consequences of reduced blood flow to the body relative to the head in an embryo that is exposed to malnutrition or hypoxia. As the arteries form and develop in such a body, they would experience lower blood pressure. Both animal studies and observations on humans have shown that arteries that develop under conditions of normal blood pressure tend to be thick-walled and elastic, whereas arteries that have been exposed to low blood pressure during their development are thin-walled and inelastic (Berry, 1978). It is a general characteristic of tissues and organs that they respond to use and increased demand ('use it or lose it'). Muscles become larger and stronger in response to work, smaller and weaker if they are not used; bones become stronger in response to increased load (within limits), and get thinner and weaker if they are not used.

● Astronauts on space missions experience no weight on their bones or normal tension in their limb muscles. How can they prevent their bones and muscles from becoming weaker during long space flights?

● They must exercise in such a way that bones and muscles experience mechanical loads, such as by isometric exercises in which one muscle is pitted against another, which puts stress on the bones to which the muscles are attached.

Most of these responses of tissues and organs in the adult are reversible. However, during the development of the embryo and the early infant, developmental processes can be diverted along pathways that have irreversible consequences, as we have seen. The formation of thin-walled, inelastic arteries under conditions of low blood pressure is one of these irreversible developments. The arteries of the adult then have reduced elasticity and this can result in susceptibility to hypertension. So a possible link is revealed between the initially quite surprising relationship that the Southampton Group discovered between the ratio of placental to baby weight and the tendency for the adults to develop high blood pressure.

This study points to health as a process that involves the conditions and experiences of an individual over the whole of a lifetime, from conception to death. Responsibility for health is not in the hands of individuals alone. It also lies with the community and with society, in ensuring adequate nutrition of its members and an absence of severe environmental stress due to such factors as air and water pollution, homelessness, unemployment and personal isolation, which can act through pregnant mothers on the embryo. The fact that there has been a significant increase in inequality in the UK since 1979 means that the health of the nation will deteriorate simply because fundamentals are being ignored. (The Income and Wealth Inquiry conducted by the Joseph Rowntree Foundation in 1995 showed that 20–30% of the population suffer social hardship.) Though well protected from a considerable range of influences, the developing person in the womb is prone to lasting damage from excessive stress, just as is an adult. The work of the Southampton Group reinforces what common sense suggests. It draws attention again to the formative period of human life, the relationship between the mother and the developing child in the womb, where the foundations of health are established. We shall return to a closer examination of the processes involved in early development in the next section of this chapter.

Summary of Section 1.5

1   Evidence for connections between environmental conditions experienced by individuals and their health can be obtained by epidemiological studies.

2   One such study suggests that malnutrition or hypoxia experienced by a developing embryo due to an inadequate diet or smoking by the mother puts the child at risk of hypertension (high blood pressure) in later life.

3   This emphasizes collective responsibility for the welfare of mothers to ensure the health of future generations.

1.6 The human body

We have looked at some of the factors that may affect our biology and health and given consideration to methods that can be used to help us understand interactions between our environment and our biology. We have yet to examine the subject of our studies – the human body.

Already you know a great deal about your own biology. Indeed, we have made a number of assumptions about your knowledge, with references to genes, blood pressure and placenta, for example, which were barely explained. As we said in Section 1.3.2, science has enormously advanced our understanding of the way the human body functions but, as this course will reveal, there is still much that we do not know. Why should that be so? Why so many mysteries?

Reflect for a moment on the photographs in Figure 1.4. One shows a sculpture by Auguste Rodin (1840–1917) entitled *The Kiss*, the other a couple in a similar pose.

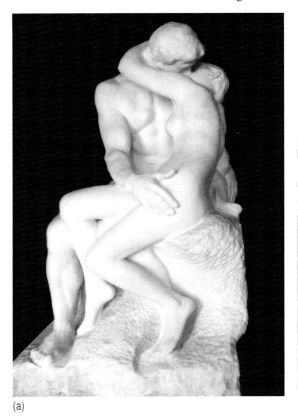

(a)

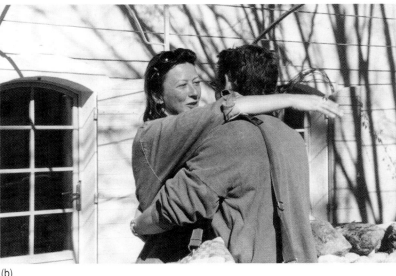

(b)

Figure 1.4   (a) *The Kiss*, a sculpture in marble by Auguste Rodin. (b) A couple in an embrace.

● Think back 100 years, then forward 100 years: now identify a key difference between the subjects of the two photographs.

○ The sculpture was created from a lump of marble over 100 years ago and in 100 years time it will (barring accidents) appear exactly as it does today. But the couple were not even born 100 years ago and in another 100 years time they will be dead.

The cycle of life encompasses birth and death and in the period between these there is growth and maintenance. What exactly does this involve? As you might imagine it involves rather more than we can hope to study in one short course! We develop from a microscopically small, single fertilized egg (known as a **zygote**). This zygote formed when a female sex cell (known as an **ovum**) was successfully fertilized by a male sex cell (known as a **sperm**). Incidentally, sex cells are known as **gametes** and there will be more about them and the whole process of reproduction in the final book of the course. You'll notice that we are assuming that you know that **cells** are the units from which all living things are made. A cell is the lowest level of biological organization capable of performing all the activities necessary to sustain independent life. If we remained as a single cell life would be a relatively straightforward affair. In fact there are many, different kinds of single-celled organisms and often school children have the opportunity of looking at a drop of pond water through a light microscope to see some of these tiny cells as they whizz or slowly glide across the field of view (Figure 1.5).

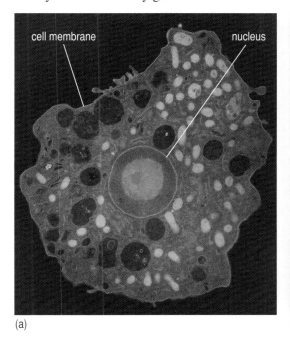

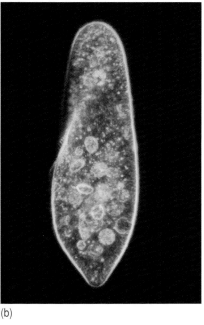

(a)   (b)

Figure 1.5   Unicellular (i.e. single-celled) pond organisms: (a) an amoeba; (b) a paramecium.

These small organisms all have a boundary layer (a bit like a 'skin') that keeps them as a discrete entity, separate from their environment. This layer is the **cell membrane** (Figure 1.5a). All cells have an outer membrane constructed to the same basic plan which we'll be examining in more detail in the next chapter. In order to whizz or glide around these organisms need a supply of energy. In fact they need energy to power a number of different processes. The processes are essentially chemical reactions and if you carried out or watched chemical reactions taking place when you were at school you will remember that they took place in special equipment, even if it was only in a glass test-tube (Figure 1.6). The reason for this is that for the desired reaction to take place the reacting chemicals need to be in close proximity to one another but separate from other chemicals. So if you want to demonstrate two different reactions you need two different sets of equipment. By the same token the cell needs to have several different bits of equipment or **organelles** so that different processes can take place concurrently. We will describe these in the next chapter, for the moment only drawing attention to the organelle known as the **nucleus** (Figure 1.5a). There is typically only one nucleus in a cell and it contains the genetic material – the DNA. Although different organelles are specialized to carry out different tasks life is simple for a single-celled organism because distances are short. So if an organelle manufactures some chemicals that will help to **digest** (break down) a food item these chemicals will not have a long journey from site of manufacture to site of use. Equally, the products of digestion which may be used

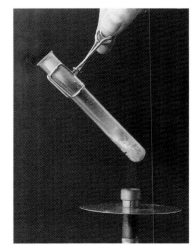

Figure 1.6   A chemical reaction taking place in a glass test-tube.

for building new cell structures or providing 'fuel' to power other cellular activities, are all going to be used within the confines of this single cell that is the organism. Contrast this with your own situation. We will examine the detail of digestion in the fourth chapter of this book but you know from experience that there is just one place where you take in food: your mouth. As some of the breakdown products are required by every cell of your body in order to 'fuel' that cell's activities, there are going to be some pretty long journeys undertaken.

Does your mouth 'water' at the mention of food? Some people find even the mere thought of a lemon or a steaming plate of curry particularly effective.

● Where do you suppose the first chemicals that help you to digest your food are found?

● They are found in your saliva. (Hence the increase in the flow of the salivary juices when you start to eat, or even to think about, food.)

In order to sustain large organisms such as ourselves it is not sufficient that there are specialized regions and organelles within each cell. Cells have to be specialized too. We are constructed from many different types of cell, each with a distinctive appearance as well as a specialized function (Figure 1.7). Our bodies are composed of **tissues**: groups of cells with a shared structure and function, associated together as a recognizable sheet, block, matrix or fluid. Examples include the muscular tissue from which our muscles are constructed, the connective tissue that binds everything together (Figure 1.8), and blood – a fluid tissue. From tissues such as these organs are composed. Organs such as the heart, brain and the salivary glands are specialized structures with distinct

Figure 1.7
(a) Photograph of a neuron (nerve cell) from the cerebral cortex of the brain. The cell bodies of other neurons can be seen in the background.
(b) Photograph of cells of the immune system (the body's defence system).

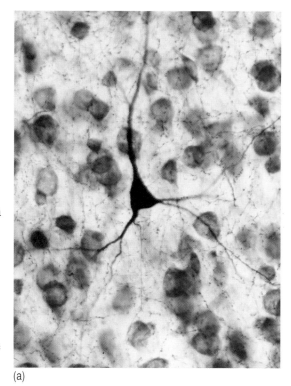
(a)

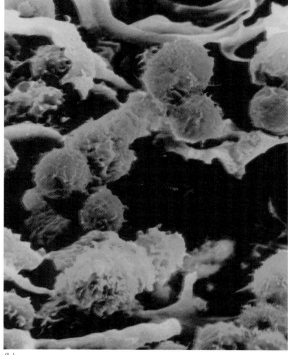
(b)

boundaries, engaged in particular functions within the body. Organs are generally composed of several different tissues, organized into very precise structures (Figure 1.9).

Organs usually work with other organs to achieve a common goal. So the salivary glands work in cooperation with other glands that produce a range of chemicals to aid digestion of your food as it passes along your gut and we refer to these organs collectively as a system: the digestive system in this case. For the sake of completeness you may wish to note that the heart is part of the cardiovascular system and the brain part of the nervous system. These systems are discussed in detail in later books but you very likely already have some idea

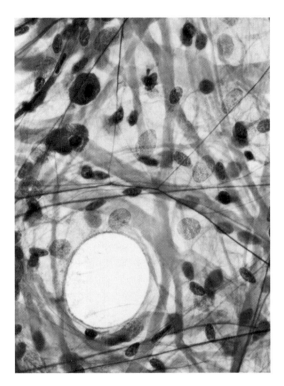

Figure 1.8   Light micrograph of areolar connective tissue. This is the most abundant connective tissue in the human body. It comprises elastin fibres (thin dark lines) and collagen fibres (thicker pink lines). Numerous cells are seen in the matrix of the tissue here, with rounded dark purple nuclei. Areolar tissue is found beneath the skin and it also links organs and other tissues.

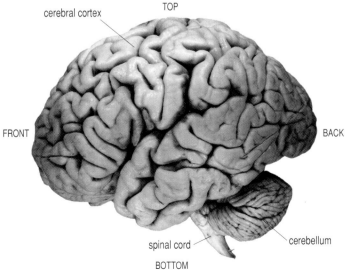

Figure 1.9   A lateral view of the human brain.

35

of their functions. One system that deserves a special mention here, because you will meet it again later in this book, although it is not discussed in detail until Book 3, is the **lymphatic system** (Figure 1.10).

Figure 1.10 The human lymphatic system, showing the primary lymphoid organs (thymus, spleen and bone marrow), the tonsils and the lymph nodes, connected by a system of lymphatic vessels and capillaries (tiny vessels). The inset of the thumb illustrates the extent of the lymphatic capillary network. *Note:* the heart and kidneys are not actually part of the lymphatic system.

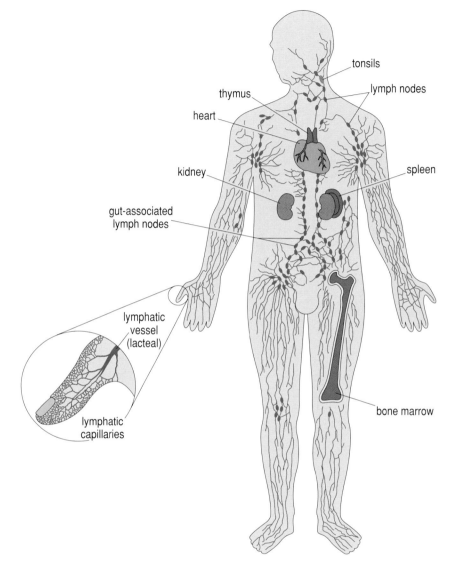

The lymphatic system consists of specialized organs, lymphatic vessels and the lymph fluid. From the inset in Figure 1.10 you can see that there is an extensive network of vessels, the lymphatic capillaries. These are closed-end vessels permeating the spaces between cells. Fluid leaks out of blood capillaries into these interstitial spaces and is then known as **interstitial fluid**. It then drains into the lymphatic capillaries (where it is called **lymph**), which eventually return it to the bloodstream via a duct connecting the lymphatic and *vascular* (blood circulatory) systems in the neck. This one-way transport system has no pump.

● Which organ is the pump for the vascular system?

● The heart.

The lymphatic system depends on the squeezing and pumping action of skeletal muscles to move fluid through its vessels. This system will be considered in more detail in Book 3, Chapter 2 but is mentioned here because it has three important functions:

1 to collect and return interstitial fluid to the blood;

2 to defend the body against invading organisms by means of the **immune system**;

3 to absorb the fatty components of your diet from the digestive tract (gut).

This last function will be considered in more detail in Chapter 4 of this book.

The lymphatic system, then, is a separate system from the cardiovascular system but clearly the two systems are functionally closely integrated, as indeed are all our body systems. There are two systems that have as their major function the role of coordinating activity within the body: the nervous system and the **endocrine system**. These two systems ensure that different parts of the body are in constant communication with each other. The **neurons** (nerve cells) of the nervous system (Figure 1.7) are responsible for transmitting and processing information, whilst **hormones** are chemicals, secreted by glands of the endocrine system, that similarly have a signalling function. One difference is that hormones are secreted into the blood and can thus circulate around the body, whilst neurons tend to communicate more intimately with other neurons or with target organs such as glands and muscles. However, although hormones circulate in the blood they only have their effects where there are cells specialized to respond to them. Both these systems are discussed in detail in Book 2. The glands that secrete hormones are known as **endocrine glands**. The salivary glands (mentioned previously) do not secrete hormones and are an example of an **exocrine gland**. Exocrine glands always have ducts along which their non-hormonal secretions pass. There are several exocrine glands associated with the digestive system.

We have moved rather swiftly from considering a single-celled organism to confronting ourselves as complex **multicellular** (many-celled) organisms. But each one of us started life as a single-celled zygote. How did we get from there to here?

In this course we are not going to give a detailed description of developmental processes, just a brief overview. Development can be defined as the collection of interrelated processes that produce a whole new individual. From this definition you might surmise that development is a life-long process, as we never stop 'developing'. For the moment we will confine ourselves to providing an overview of the stages from zygote to the birth of the baby. The study of development has a relatively short history. Until the late 17th century it was believed that a new individual was entirely preformed in the sex cells of its male parent. Indeed, some scientists of the day claimed that by using microscopes, invented in the early 17th century, they could actually see tiny preformed people – called *homunculi* – in sperm cells (Figure 1.11a, overleaf). The female was thought to act only as an oven in which the baby could grow (Figure 1.11b) until it was large enough to survive birth. However, the advent of better microscopes did not substantiate these claims, and gradually it became clear that both sperm and an egg, produced by the mother, were needed to make a baby.

Figure 1.11 (a) Homunculi claimed to be visible in sperm. (b) Pregnancy simplified and stylized. (From late 17th-century illustrations.)

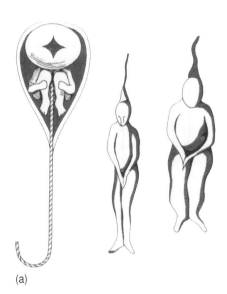

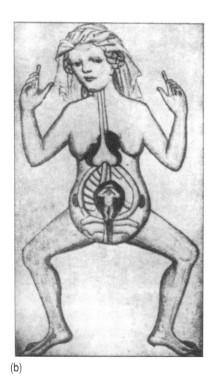

(a)   (b)

For the first week the early embryo is the same size as the zygote but the number of cells it contains is rapidly increasing.

● How can there be more cells if the embryo is not increasing in size?

● As the number of cells increases each individual cell must be smaller.

This is exactly what happens. The zygote first divides into two cells; each of these 'daughter' cells is half the size of the zygote. Three rounds of cell division result in an 8-celled embryo whose cells are all in contact with the 'outside', i.e. the fluid in the mother's womb. But the fourth division is different and, as you will see, vital for further development. The division from 8 to 16 cells is *asymmetric*, that is, the division does not occur across the centre of the cell, but is closer to one end than the other.

● What is the consequence of this asymmetry?

● The resulting cells are of two different sizes (Figure 1.12).

At the 16-cell stage, the first differentiative event has occurred: there are two populations of cells: eight large cells on the outside, and eight smaller cells on the inside. Size is not the only difference between them; the cells' membranes and constituents are different (e.g. the number of organelles in each cell might differ).

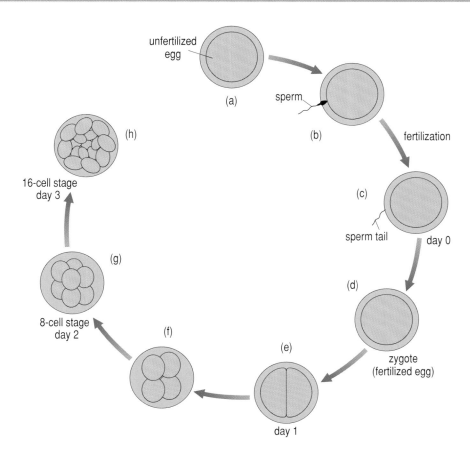

unfertilized egg

(a)

sperm

(b)

fertilization

(c)

sperm tail

day 0

(d)

zygote (fertilized egg)

(e)

day 1

(f)

8-cell stage day 2

(g)

16-cell stage day 3

(h)

Figure 1.12 The stages of early human development.

● Could these differences be attributed simply to unequal division?

◐ If the constituents of the dividing cell are shared between two daughter cells then unequal division could lead to the larger daughter cell having more constituents than the smaller cell; or even having some constituents that the smaller cell does not have. But the cell membrane cannot be simply divided in to two portions; there would not be enough 'material'. (If you wrap two paperback novels together to give to a friend you use less wrapping paper than if you take the same two books and wrap each separately.) So more cell membrane *must* be made and thus differences in cell membrane could be the result of differences in manufacture, rather than a consequence of unequal division.

In fact, one of the differences between the two types of cell is that the smaller cells are more adhesive than the larger cells and they form a tight ball of cells lying within the shell formed by the larger, outer cells. The adhesiveness is a property of some of the newly manufactured components of their cell membranes. In the next chapter we will be saying more about the processes that lead to the manufacture of these cell components but for now we will just note that it is your genetic material (DNA) that directs these operations. However, there is a paradox. Every cell of your body contains the same genetic material (your DNA 'fingerprint' which is unique to you), so how is it that, at this early stage of development, the DNA of one cell is making something different to the DNA of a sister cell?

● Can you suggest an answer to this paradox?

(Hint: we talked earlier of interaction between genes and environment (Section 1.2) and also stated that the DNA is contained in the nucleus, i.e. in an organelle that is separate from the rest of the constituents of the cell.)

● Each cell has one nucleus with identical DNA but the cellular environments are no longer identical once a few cell divisions have taken place. So by now the DNA must be interacting with its local environment (namely the cell constituents) in different ways.

So right at the start of development, before the embryo is attached to the womb, long before the mother has any idea that she might be pregnant, there are differential interactions taking place between genes and environment. The particular cellular environment in which the nucleus finds itself affects **gene expression**. We say that a gene is being expressed when it is active. Some genes – those responsible for the cell's 'house-keeping' functions, such as providing a source of energy – are expressed in all the cells of your body, while the expression of others is tissue-specific – genes that are switched on in one tissue are suppressed in others.

Around the time of the 8- to 16-cell division, the developing embryo undergoes a **morphological** (shape) change, in which the cells flatten on each other, and the outlines of individual cells become hard to distinguish. It is not possible to see the two different cell types present in a developing embryo at the 16-cell stage, although we have shown it schematically in Figure 1.12. The larger outer cells will not form part of the new individual. They form the embryo's contribution to the placenta (Figure 1.13). This organ, created in cooperation with maternal tissues, supplies nutrients and oxygen to, and removes waste products from, the embryo throughout the rest of gestation, i.e. the period of time spent in the womb (uterus). The blood circulation systems are the supply lines; maternal and fetal (**fetus** is the term used to describe the developing human after the eighth week of gestation, when all the systems of the body have been formed) circulation remain separate from one another but their blood vessels lie in close proximity to facilitate the interchange of substances. The inner cell mass becomes the new individual through processes of growth and differentiation, remaining within the safe environment of the mother's womb for around 38 weeks. During this time it is kept at an appropriate temperature, supplied with oxygen and nutrients that provide the raw materials for growth and has its waste products removed.

● What happens to the placenta if the mother's diet is inadequate?

● The placenta grows larger, increasing the area of intimate contact with the mother's circulation, thereby attempting to scavenge more of the available nutrients from the maternal blood vessels (Section 1.5).

● Why do you think mothers are advised against alcohol and other drugs/medication during pregnancy?

● There is the potential for any substance found in the mother's blood to pass to the developing fetus.

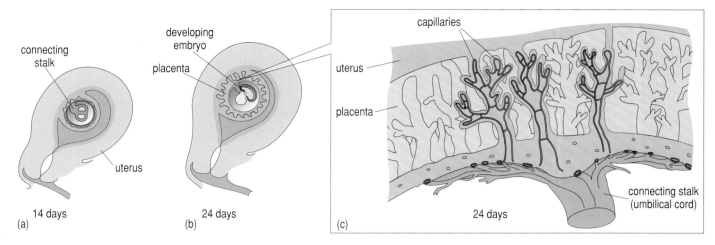

Figure 1.13 The gross changes that occur in the form of the early embryo are shown schematically (a and b), illustrating the growth of the placenta (c).

Mention has already been made of the existence of sensitive periods during development of rats (Section 1.5.2); there are also known sensitive periods during human development.

● From general knowledge, can you name one infectious disease that can cause damage to the human embryo in the first three months of pregnancy?

● The German measles, or rubella, virus can pass from mother to baby across the placenta.

If this happens during the first three months of pregnancy it can seriously damage the embryo, leading to **congenital** abnormalities such as deafness or blindness, even death. Congenital means a condition that the baby is born with: it includes, but is not limited to, inherited conditions.

Although the rubella virus can easily pass across the placenta, as can alcohol, nicotine and some other substances, in general the barrier of a few layers of cells between the blood vessels of the mother and those of the embryo provides an effective screen for the embryo against harmful agents, such as disease-causing organisms, that might be in the mother's blood. The placenta does a marvellous job of protecting the embryo from these agents.

The embryo grows on in the mother's womb, totally dependent on the mother for all its needs, until at birth it is pushed out into a hostile world to lead a semi-independent life. In order to be able to live independently of its mother there are a number of changes that have to be made to the new baby's physiology as well as to the way it behaves.

● Can you give one example of a change that must occur as soon as the baby is born as a consequence of the baby now finding itself surrounded by air rather than the watery fluid in which it was previously suspended?

● The baby has been getting oxygen from its mother's blood but it must now take air into its lungs and extract oxygen from the air.

In the chapter on circulation in Book 3 we'll find out how this transformation works and learn about some structural changes that have to take place at birth to ensure the new system works efficiently. Big changes take place at birth but not all systems are immediately fully mature and functional. The new-born is vulnerable and you'll discover in this course how systems change and mature through life. Most reach peak performance after around 20 years of life, then, sadly, decline. But we have tremendous reserve capacity in most body systems. For example, we can continue to function adequately with only one kidney. We are aware that muscle output and cognitive activity often decline with age but we can actually do a great deal to keep body systems in good condition.

Summary of Section 1.6

1   The individual develops from a single-celled zygote into a complex multicellular being.

2   Cells become differentiated and form a variety of tissues, organs and organ systems.

1.7 Looking forward

Before we look at individual systems we need to introduce the basic chemical and biological background necessary to understand the development and functioning of the human body. We will do this in the next chapter and it will be necessary to take a reductionist perspective when studying this basic science. Yet our aim is to retain the holistic perspective throughout this course and a major tool will be the case reports that appear in every chapter. Whilst the diseases show-cased in these reports will relate to the systems currently under discussion the reports should serve to remind you that individuals are not just a collection of systems. The importance of considering interactions between systems and in particular the emotional impact when treating or supporting someone with a disease will be evident from these accounts of the experience of real people.

Questions for Chapter 1

Question 1.1 (Learning Outcome 1.1)

Summarize in two paragraphs the main strengths and weaknesses of reductionist and holistic approaches to researching the influences on health.

Question 1.2 (LO 1.2)

Identical twins have identical genes. What would a person who believes in biological determinism predict about the growth and development of identical twins who were separated at birth and brought up by different families?

Question 1.3 (LO 1.3)

The Inuit people of the Arctic circle have small pads of fat around their eye sockets, which push the eyelids forward, so that they cover more of the eyeball than is the case in people who live in more temperate climates. It has been argued that these pads help to protect the eyes from the damaging brilliance of a snow-bound landscape.

How would the evolution of the fat pads be explained by an evolutionary biologist? Include the following terms in your answer: natural selection; adaptive characteristic; survival advantage; fitness; evolution.

Question 1.4 (LO 1.4)

It could be claimed that epidemiological studies are of no value in the study of disease because they are unable to identify specific causes. What is your view on this?

Question 1.5 (LO 1.5)

Suppose that a friend of yours who is pregnant and also a heavy smoker has heard that smoking tends to reduce the baby's weight thus making the delivery easier and safer. What would be your advice to her?

References

Armstrong, D. (1986) The problem of the whole person in holistic medicine, *Holistic Medicine*, **1**, 27–36. (An edited version appears in Davey, B., Gray, A. and Seale, C. (eds) (1995) *Health and Disease: A Reader*, 2nd edn, Buckingham: Open University Press.)

Barker, D. J. P. (1992) *Fetal and Infant Origins of Adult Disease*. Cambridge: Tavistock Press.

Barker, D. J. P., Bull, A. R., Osmond, C. and Simmonds, S. J. (1990) Fetal and placental size and risk of hypertension in adult life, *British Medical Journal*, **301**, 259–262.

Berry, C. L. (1978) Hypertension and arterial development: long-term considerations, *British Heart Journal*, **40**, 709–717.

Dawkins, R. (1976) *The Selfish Gene*. Oxford: Oxford University Press.

Department of Health (2001) *The Expert Patient: a new approach to chronic disease management*. London: Department of Health.

Hills, J. (1995) *Joseph Rowntree Foundation Inquiry into Income and Wealth, Vol. 2: A summary of the evidence*. York: Joseph Rowntree Foundation.

World Health Organization (1958) *Constitution of the World Health Organization*, Annex 1, Geneva.

CHAPTER 2

WONDERFUL LIFE

Learning Outcomes

After completing this chapter, you should be able to:

2.1 Outline how the basic principles of atomic structure and chemical bonding affect the structure and function of the molecular constituents of living organisms.

2.2 Explain how living organisms are able to maintain homeostasis by holding regulated variables within specified limits through a mix of negative feedback and feedforward control systems.

2.3 Describe and understand the roles of the various subcellular structures.

2.4 Describe the processes underlying gene expression.

2.5 Outline the nuclear and chromosomal events that occur during mitosis and demonstrate an understanding of how these relate to the development of cancer.

2.6 Give an account of the stages of wound healing and the basic processes involved in restoring the integrity of the tissues.

2.1 Introduction

'...*ashes to ashes, dust to dust...*'

Being alive is an extraordinary state to be in. Indeed life seems so amazing and improbable that for centuries a 'life force' was postulated. Without this 'life force' the human body (or any other organism) returned to the dust from which it was assumed to have sprung. With the 'life force' life could be created from a handful of dust. Hence the lines from the *Book of Common Prayer* that are quoted at the start of this chapter. Of course, by the time the *Book of Common Prayer* was written, no-one was thinking literally in terms of individuals being created from handfuls of dust, although to this day there continue to be interesting debates about when a new *individual* comes into being. (These can be approached from philosophical, psychological, religious and sociological viewpoints, as well as from the biological, and will be touched upon in Book 4.) However, it is remarkable that, at one level, the material from which we are made is no different to the material from which the sculpture shown in Figure 1.4 is made. Everything around you right now, the walls of the room, the chair you are sitting in, the book in front of you, the air you breathe – in fact all matter – is made up of collections of individual particles called **atoms**.

2.2 Constituents of matter

2.2.1 Atoms and elements

In high power photographs such as Figure 2.1 atoms have the appearance of solid spheres. This is illusory, for experimental evidence shows that they are made from several different sub-atomic particles and a lot of empty space. They have a core containing two types of particles which are named neutrons and **protons**. Around this central cluster of particles are negatively charged particles called **electrons,** arranged in successive layers. The electrons in an atom circle fast and unpredictably around the centre, forming a cloud of negative **charge**; these clouds are usually represented in diagrams as circles (Figure 2.2). Charge is a concept that will crop up frequently in this course. In everyday life we come across the term when discussing electrical equipment. So you may have talked about 'charging up' your car battery or mobile phone. Charge obviously has something to do with providing electrical energy in these contexts. The way we are using it here is not so very different. In addition to electric current or 'moving' electricity you may be familiar with the idea of static (non-moving) electricity. The effects of static electricity are seen when objects such as hair or clothing acquire a charge. This comes about because atoms can lose electrons. For example, brushing hair can result in electrons being lost from the hair and transferring to the brush. The objects that have this electric charge do not look any different from before, but they do react with other objects differently. For instance, hair may have a 'fly away' look as similarly charged hairs repel each other. The only way you can tell that something is charged is to see how it reacts with other charged objects. An object can have a positive charge or a negative charge, or it can be uncharged.

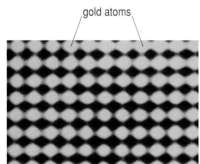

gold atoms

Figure 2.1 A thin layer of gold, in which the atoms appear as bright spots. The atoms are about 10^{-10} (i.e. 0.000 000 000 1) centimetres (cm) apart.

● An atom is uncharged. It is formed of uncharged neutrons, negatively charged electrons and of protons. What can you deduce about the state of protons?

○ Protons must be positively charged to counteract the negative charge of the electrons and thus leave the atom as an uncharged particle.

Each proton has an equal and opposite charge to each electron. So an uncharged atom has equal numbers of protons and electrons. The atom does not have an electric charge overall because the positive and negative charges cancel each other.

We have just said that objects with the same charge (such as electrostatically charged hairs) repel each other. Those with opposite charges, one positive and one negative, attract each other. The positively charged protons in the nucleus of the atom attract and hold the negatively charged electrons. The term charge therefore is used to describe the property of some objects that is responsible for electrostatic interactions between them.

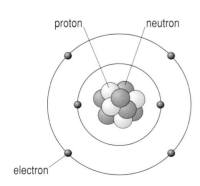

proton   neutron

electron

Figure 2.2 Simplified structure of an atom of carbon.

● Suppose an electron were to be attracted away from its atom. In terms of charge how would you now describe the atom?

○ If an electron were removed from the atom it would take with it one unit of negative charge and leave the 'atom' as a positively charged particle.

Similarly, if the atom were to obtain an extra electron and add it to the cloud of negative charge around it, the 'atom' would become a negatively charged particle. This can happen and these 'charged atoms' are called **ions**. They are very important for biological activity and we shall come across mention of them in many chapters of this course.

Figure 2.2 shows the structure of just one particular type of atom – a carbon atom. All carbon atoms have six protons and six neutrons in the inner core and the positive charge of the protons is balanced by six electrons. The structure of an oxygen atom or a nitrogen atom is different.

Carbon, oxygen and nitrogen are each examples of **elements**. Elements are defined as substances that contain only one type of atom; put another way, atoms of different elements differ from one another in their atomic structure, i.e. in the number of neutrons, protons and electrons from which they are made. There are 92 naturally occurring elements, but living matter uses only a small proportion of these. In fact, organisms are made largely out of just four elements: carbon, hydrogen, oxygen and nitrogen. Oxygen, nitrogen and hydrogen exist as gases in the Earth's atmosphere. Nitrogen is the most abundant (making up about 80% of the air) and hydrogen the least abundant (less than 1%). Oxygen makes up about 20% of the air and is the element involved in burning – all methods used to extinguish fires involve excluding oxygen. As you will see later, oxygen fulfils a similar and vital role in the cells of living organisms in the 'burning' of food to provide energy.

● From general knowledge can you think of elements other than the four just mentioned that are found in living matter like ourselves?

◌ Calcium is needed for strong bones and teeth; iron is needed for the proper functioning of blood.

In addition, sodium and chlorine, the two elements from which table salt (sodium chloride) is composed, are needed for proper nerve and muscle function. Other elements such as the metals zinc, selenium, cobalt, chromium and copper are required by the body in very small amounts and are therefore called **trace elements**. Many of these trace elements are poisonous if consumed in quantities significantly larger than those occurring naturally in the diet. That this is so has been known for a long while and has provided the core of the plot for many 'murder–mystery' novels where the cunning of the murderer in finding a 'natural' way of dispatching their victim was offset by the skill of the detective well versed in the signs and symptoms of such poisons.

2.2.2 Chemical compounds

Each element is represented by a one- or two-letter symbol. As these are often used as a form of 'short-hand' you will find it useful to recognize those for the main elements found in living matter. However, elements are not commonly found in their pure form but in combination with each other to form **compounds**. Compounds are substances composed of two or more elements, i.e. types of atom. The most abundant compound in living matter (and indeed on Earth) is water, accounting for an average of 60% of total human body weight. Water is a compound of the gaseous elements hydrogen and oxygen. The symbol for hydrogen is H, the symbol for oxygen is O. Water is represented by the symbols H_2O.

● What do you suppose the subscript '2' tells you about the way that hydrogen has combined with oxygen to form water?

● You might already know, or have guessed correctly, that it means that two atoms of hydrogen combine with one atom of oxygen to form one 'unit' of water.

The processes in which different combinations of elements are made or destroyed are called chemical reactions. When chemical reactions take place in cells they are called **metabolic processes**. The properties of compounds are often very different from those of their constituent elements. For example, oxygen and hydrogen are gases whereas water is a liquid.

Atoms can form stable interactions with other atoms by sharing electrons. When electrons are shared to form a stable 'unit' we call the unit a **molecule** and we say that the shared electrons have formed a **covalent bond**. Atoms can share one pair of electrons between them to give a single bond. In Figure 2.3 you can see how water is formed; note the two single bonds. When atoms share two pairs of electrons this is called a **double bond**.

Figure 2.3   The formation of a water molecule. Note that each atom of oxygen shares one pair of electrons with the hydrogen atom. The stable water molecule therefore has two single bonds.

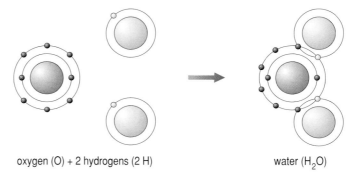

oxygen (O) + 2 hydrogens (2 H)   water (H$_2$O)

● You have already come across another way that atoms can be made stable. In the previous section we described how electrons might be attracted away from, or added to an atom. What was the name of the particle so formed?

● When an atom gains or loses electrons it becomes an ion.

Table salt (sodium chloride) is another example of a stable compound. It is formed from the elements sodium and chlorine. The two elements, sodium and chlorine, combine together by forming ions (charged particles) as shown in Figure 2.4. The sodium ion has a positive charge and is represented symbolically by Na$^+$, and the chlor*ide* (not chlor*ine*, now that it's in a compound) as Cl$^-$.

Figure 2.4   Formation of sodium chloride. An atom of sodium donates a single electron to a chlorine atom, thereby becoming a positively charged sodium ion. The chlorine atom becomes a negatively charged chloride ion.

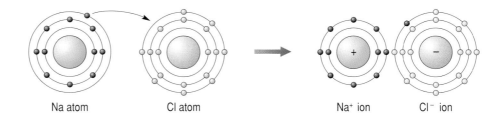

Na atom   Cl atom   Na$^+$ ion   Cl$^-$ ion

- In what ratio (proportion) do the elements of sodium and chlorine combine when forming sodium chloride? (Look at Figure 2.4 to work out the answer.)

- One atom of sodium reacts with one atom of chlorine to form a stable compound, so the ratio is 1:1.

This is represented symbolically as NaCl. NaCl is known as the **molecular formula** of sodium chloride. The molecular formula therefore tells you not only which elements have combined to form a compound but also in what ratio they have combined.

- What is the molecular formula for water?

- The molecular formula for water is H_2O.

- In Figure 2.4 the Na^+ ion has a positive charge and the Cl^- a negative charge. How then do they interact with each other to maintain a stable compound?

- Na^+ and Cl^- are held together by their opposite electrical charges.

This is an example of **ionic bonding**.

Atoms combine to form compounds using bonds that are either covalent or ionic. The type of bonds that will be used depends on the nature of the atoms of the elements involved.

Summary of Section 2.2

1   Matter is made up of particles called atoms.

2   An atom has a central core comprising neutrons and positively charged protons. Negatively charged electrons encircle the central core.

3   An atom that acquires extra electrons or loses electrons becomes a charged particle called an ion.

4   An element contains only one type of atom.

5   The trace elements are those required by the body in very small amounts.

6   Elements combine with each other to form compounds.

7   The chemical reactions that take place in the body are collectively called metabolic processes.

8   Covalent compounds are made up of discrete molecules that share electrons, forming covalent bonds; ionic compounds form when ions are held together by the attraction of their opposite electrical charges, resulting in ionic bonds.

2.3 The chemistry of life

We often talk about the chemistry between two people. An acknowledgement perhaps of the way that two discrete individuals can react with one another to form a relationship that is more than the sum of its parts in a process analogous to the chemical reaction between two elements that results in a compound with properties quite distinct from those of either element. Or it may be that we are acknowledging the extraordinary fact that we are constructed from the same particles as all earthly matter and that the metabolic processes that occur in our bodies and underpin all living processes; from growth to reproduction, are subject to exactly the same laws and constraints as any other chemical process or reaction. All this is true but there is something that is distinctive about the chemistry of life. Life is carbon based. The molecules that make up living things range in size from the very small, such as the water molecule, to extremely large molecules, such as DNA. (Very large molecules are called **macromolecules**.) All biological macromolecules contain carbon. Carbon atoms can form numerous varied molecular structures, many more than can any other element. They can form long chains, join with many different elements and form ring structures. The study of the chemistry of carbon compounds forms a specialized branch of chemistry known as **organic** chemistry. Substances that do not contain carbon are referred to as inorganic. (The term 'organic' is a relic of the days when chemists thought that these compounds were derived only from living matter – *organisms* – or from matter that was once living. It was subsequently discovered that organic molecules could be made from non-living matter.) Now that you know the meaning of the word 'organic' it may seem to you incredible that any one could conceive of calling a vegetable or a chicken anything other than 'organic'! This is just one of many examples you will have to contend with, where the scientific meaning of a word differs from its everyday definition. Another example you might have noticed in passing was 'element', which bears no comparison with the electric 'element' in your kettle or the expression, 'braving the elements' which usually means that you are about to go out into the wind and rain!

2.3.1 The macromolecules

There are four types of macromolecule: carbohydrates, lipids (fats), proteins and nucleic acids. Each macromolecule is composed of a number of smaller, component molecules: proteins, for example, are composed of **amino acids**. The component molecules are all obtained from the diet. Usually, whatever food is eaten, it is in the form of macromolecules, which have to be broken down (i.e. digested) into their chemical components. These are then transported in the bloodstream to cells, where they are metabolized, i.e. converted into other chemical components or assembled into the macromolecules and structures of your own body.

A few chemicals, e.g. water and salt, are obtained directly from the diet, i.e. they enter the body directly without needing to be broken down and reassembled.

Carbohydrates and lipids require only a brief word here; they will be defined and explored more fully in Chapter 3. Carbohydrates such as starch can be broken down to their chemical components, one of which is the crucial energy-yielding molecule **glucose**. Cells that have high energy demands, such as those in the brain, the nervous system, and muscles need to be supplied with lots of glucose. Lipids (fatty substances) are present in large quantities in cell membranes. Both carbohydrates, stored as glycogen, and lipids, (all too easily) stored as fat in **adipose tissue**, can be utilized at a later time as an energy source.

Proteins need to be considered in more detail than do carbohydrates or lipids. Proteins are important for a number of reasons; for example, certain proteins, called **enzymes**, control metabolic processes. The enzymes dictate which chemical conversions can occur, and hence which chemical constituents can be made. A simple example will illustrate the point. Most animals have the enzymes necessary to convert glucose into vitamin C. However, we do not have the appropriate enzymes in our cells, so we cannot make vitamin C from glucose – a failing we share with other primates and with guinea pigs. (Vitamin C is essential for life, so we must obtain vitamin C directly from the diet.) Enzymes and other proteins are considered further in Section 2.3.2.

Nucleic acids also need to be considered in more detail. We have already met one nucleic acid, deoxyribo*nucleic acid* (DNA). DNA, is found in the cell nucleus, and comprises the genetic material. DNA is the chemical component of the long-term information stores more usually referred to as genes. The other nucleic acid, ribo*nucleic acid*, **RNA**, serves a number of functions, one of which is as a short-term information store, relaying information from the nucleus to the rest of the cell. This important function determines which proteins are to be assembled in the cell at any one moment. DNA contains the full complement of an organism's genes and, it is the genes that determine which proteins an organism has. We do not have the proteins, the enzymes, needed to make vitamin C, because we do not have the necessary genes. The structure and function of DNA is considered in Sections 2.6 and 2.7.

2.3.2 Proteins and enzymes

Proteins have many and varied functions, all of which are necessary for life. Some proteins are contractile. Muscle, for instance, consists principally of the proteins **actin** and **myosin**. Some proteins contribute to the shape of individual cells and structures (e.g. blood vessels and heart). Others act as messengers in the organism, being released from cells in one part of the body and affecting the activity of cells in another part of the body. **Insulin**, for example, is a hormone that is released from the pancreas and assists the uptake of glucose from the bloodstream into the cells. Some proteins are **receptors** that detect these messengers. They are situated in the membranes of cells and when they are activated by messengers such as insulin they alter the properties of the membrane allowing the entry or exit of ions or molecules and thereby influencing the cells activities. (Receptor is a term used to describe any part of our body that detects what is going on around it. So we also call groups of cells that are responsive to sensory events in the world around us receptors, such as the **photoreceptors**, the light-sensitive receptor cells found in the cell layer known as the **retina** of the eye.)

Every species of living organism has its own characteristic set of proteins, called the *proteome*. Humans can make somewhere between 50 000 and 70 000 different proteins in total. Some of these proteins are very similar or even identical to those of other organisms, but only humans have the human proteome. That does not mean that all the cells of your body produce all these proteins all the time; far from it. You produce a different subset of the proteome at different times during your life. Furthermore, different tissues produce different subsets of the proteome from each other. It does appear that proteins are made to order; so that the right protein is in the right tissues at the right time. The way in which protein production is controlled is a key element of change in all its forms, i.e. growth, development, healing, reproduction as well as behaviours that are characteristic of our mental life such as learning and memory. Section 2.7 describes protein production.

Proteins are made of amino acids joined one to another into strings. Short strings, of up to ten amino acids, are sometimes called **peptides**, whilst longer strings are called **polypeptides**. Biochemists use the terms 'protein' and 'polypeptide' rather loosely and interchangeably. Here too both terms are used. Twenty or so different amino acids are commonly found in living organisms and, in various combinations, they make up the proteins found in our bodies. By arranging different numbers of amino acids in different orders, so different proteins can be made. (It is worth noting that if you wished to make a string of only six amino acids there are 64 million different ways in which this could be configured! The number of possible proteins is therefore enormous.) The exact order in which the amino acids are joined together, known as the primary structure of the protein, is dictated by the genetic material by means of the genetic code (Section 2.7).

However, a protein is not simply a string of amino acids: a protein has a unique three-dimensional shape (Figure 2.5). The shape arises because a particular string of amino acids folds up on itself in a particular way. The shape is then held stable by chemical bonding between specific amino acids. The precise shape of a protein is often decisive in the functioning of that protein: if the protein is the wrong shape, its functioning will be impaired, or worse, it will not function at all. A mistake in joining the amino acids together into a string, so that just one is of the wrong kind or in the wrong place or missing, can alter the shape of the folded protein and result in a protein which simply cannot do its job. It is therefore, literally, vital that proteins are made accurately.

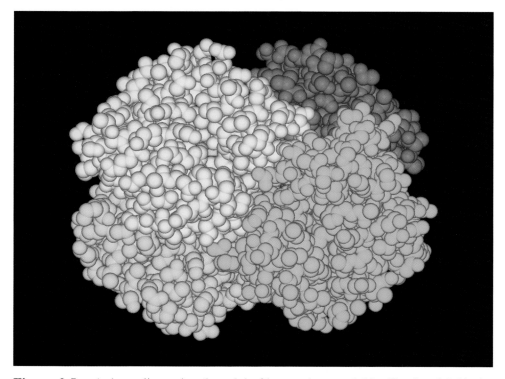

Figure 2.5 A three-dimensional model of human haemoglobin (Section 2.3.3), the protein in red blood cells that carries oxygen. The four subunits of the protein are coloured differently in this representation. The subunits are formed from four strings of amino acids (polypeptides) which then aggregate to give the globular structure shown here.

Enzymes, one particular sort of protein, control the rates at which the myriad chemical conversions in cells take place; most chemical conversions in cells would be very slow, or would not occur at all without enzymes. (Enzymes are very specific *catalysts*: each one speeds up a chemical reaction without itself undergoing any net change in the process.) Enzymes do, however, require very precise working conditions. If they are overheated or if their environment is too acid they *denature*, i.e. their three-dimensional structure crumbles and they fall apart.

Cells producing a particular subset of the proteome are said to be specialized.

● In Chapter 1 we observed that cells start to differentiate (i.e. specialize) early in development. When is this differentiation first seen?

● The first sign of differentiation is at the 16-cell stage, two days after fertilization has occurred.

● Why is specialization necessary?

● Large organisms such as ourselves must have specialized cells and organ systems to convey information and materials to all parts of the body.

For example, a cell may be specialized to produce and release insulin into the bloodstream. To do so it must contain the molecular machinery to synthesize insulin, to secrete insulin and to control both of these processes in response to signals from elsewhere in the body. Other cells may be specialized to produce **myelin**, the fat-rich electrically insulating sheath which surrounds some neurons, whilst others may be the neurons themselves. However, humans do not produce cells specialized in the production of silk; nor do spiders have specialized cells to produce the fat-rich electrically insulating sheath of myelin which surrounds neurons. The reason for these differences lies in the DNA of humans and spiders, respectively. We will consider this remarkable molecule in Sections 2.7 and 2.8.

2.3.3 Water

Although life is carbon-based there is another compound that is crucial for life: a small inorganic molecule. As you have probably guessed on account of the fact that it constitutes about 60% of your body weight, the molecule is water. Water is incredibly useful because so many substances dissolve in it. Once the substance has dissolved in water the result is referred to as a solution. Water is not the only fluid that can act as a solvent so when any substance is dissolved in water it is called an aqueous solution (from the Latin *aqua* meaning water). In any solution the solvent is the substance that is present in the greater amount and is pretty much unaltered in its physical and chemical state. The substance that is dissolved (known as the solute) eventually becomes evenly dispersed throughout the solution. We say that the substance is moving down its **concentration gradient**. This process is called **diffusion**. Diffusion is an important process for it enables some substances to move between different body fluids, as you will shortly read (Section 2.5.1). It is, however, a relatively slow process.

● There is a common household substance whose molecular formula you now know that dissolves in water. What is its common name, its chemical name and its molecular formula?

● Table salt (sodium chloride, NaCl) dissolves in water.

Figure 2.6a shows the structure of solid salt; note how the ions of Na^+ and Cl^- are held together in a crystal lattice by ionic bonds. The ionic bonds are very strong and it takes very high temperatures to supply enough energy to prise the bonds apart so that the substance turns into a liquid, i.e. melts (Figure 2.6b). In the liquid the ions are mobile.

● If salt dissolves in water can the ions remain in their lattice formation?

● No. In solution the salt is evenly dispersed through the solution so the ions must have become mobile.

● If you place a small amount of salt in water will it dissolve without being heated?

● Yes it will. (It will dissolve more quickly if you heat it but it certainly does not require the very high temperatures that are needed to melt solid salt.)

This means that water must have some remarkable ability that enables it to prise the ions apart. It does! Water molecules surround each ion of Na^+ and Cl^- forming a 'shell' – the ions are then said to be solvated. With a shell of water molecules around them the electrostatic forces, attracting the positively charged sodium and the negatively charged chloride ions to one another, are weakened and the solvated ions are free to move further apart (Figure 2.6c). In fact it is these charges on the ions that attract the water molecules in the first place and causes them to surround each ion. This is very strange given that we have just explained that water molecules are formed from hydrogen and oxygen by the

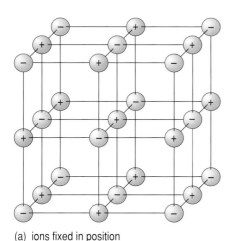

(a) ions fixed in position

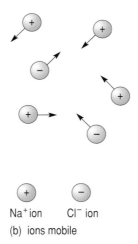

Na^+ ion Cl^- ion

(b) ions mobile

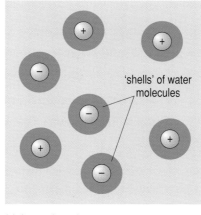

'shells' of water molecules

(c) ions solvated

Figure 2.6 (a) Lattice structure of a crystal of sodium chloride (NaCl) – as a solid the ions are fixed in space. (b) Liquid (molten) NaCl – the ions are mobile. (c) Solvated Na^+ and Cl^- ions in aqueous solution.

sharing of electrons (covalent bonding), hence there is no overall charge on the water molecules. So why are they attracted to the Na^+ and Cl^- ions? It turns out that although some atoms do share electrons equally when they form covalent bonds others don't. Some atoms pull electrons toward their central mass very strongly. In the case of the water molecule, the oxygen atom pulls more of the electrons towards it, giving it a partial negative charge, whilst the hydrogen atoms now have a partial positive charge. The bond holding the water molecule together is therefore not uniform. It has a positive end and a negative end. When a structure has ends that differ in some way such as this we often use the term polar. (The Earth has a North Pole and a South Pole; when people hold different views they can be described as polarized views). So covalent bonds that have a polarity are called **polar covalent bonds**.

Many substances dissolve in water due to solvation. In fact, water is essential to life because it dissolves and holds many different substances in the same liquid. Substances may be held in solution to facilitate their transport from place to place. For example, blood is a water-based tissue. It contains red and white blood cells in a yellowish, watery **plasma**. Plasma is 90% water and (amongst other things) carries dissolved gases such as oxygen. (Blood is not able to hold sufficient oxygen in solution to meet the needs of all the body's cells but the protein haemoglobin (from the Greek *haima*, 'blood' and *globin* for its globular structure; Figure 2.5) carries higher concentrations of oxygen within red blood cells – more details will be given in Book 3.) Importantly, solvation facilitates reactions between different ions. This allows the chemical reactions that are the basis for all living processes to occur. In the next section we review these processes and identify the characteristics that are distinctive of metabolic as opposed to any other kind of chemical reaction.

Summary of Section 2.3

1   Life is based on carbon-containing (organic) compounds. Substances that do not contain carbon are referred to as inorganic.

2   Very large molecules are called macromolecules. The four types of macromolecules, carbohydrate, lipids (fats), proteins and nucleic acids, are formed from component molecules that are obtained from our diet.

3   Carbohydrates and lipids are an important energy source.

4   Nucleic acids (DNA and RNA) compose genes (DNA) and relay instructions for making proteins (RNA).

5   Proteins have structural, hormonal, defence, transport and catalytic (enzymatic) roles. The proteome is an organism's set of proteins.

6   Proteins are macromolecules made up of combinations of 20 amino acid building blocks.

7   The primary structure of a protein determines its three-dimensional structure and shape which in turn determines its function.

8   Water is essential for life as so many substances can dissolve in it.

9   Polar covalent bonds are so called because the electrons are not shared equally, so the bond has a negative end and a positive end.

2.4 What is life?

The distinctive feature of metabolic processes in living organisms is the way in which they are organized. Living organisms:

- are self-regulating.
- direct their own metabolic processes.

Growth, repair and reproduction all occur as a consequence of metabolic processes that are directed by genes. Energy is required for these activities, just as for any other chemical synthesis. Our energy needs are met from the food we eat but the process of obtaining that energy from our diet does not contravene any of the 'laws' of chemical reactions. In metabolizing dietary items, both to provide energy and for the production of building blocks for growth and repair, waste products will be created and these are ultimately **excreted** (eliminated from the body) mostly in the urine. (Waste material that is not digested passes through the length of the gut and is voided from the anus. This is **defaecation** not excretion. Excretion only refers to substances that have been incorporated into the body.) The process that provides energy using oxygen (from the air) and glucose (from food) is **respiration** (more correctly: aerobic respiration – *aerobic* meaning 'oxygen using'– because you will later discover that energy can be supplied for a short time without using oxygen). Respiration is the chemical process that takes place in every cell, so sometimes it is called cellular respiration. We obtain the glucose by eating and the oxygen by breathing. When we breathe out (exhale), the air has not only had some oxygen removed from it, it has had a waste gas called carbon dioxide added to it. So this process can also be described as a form of excretion.

All the metabolic processes necessary for life can take place in a single cell. An essential requirement is that the cellular environment must be kept within prescribed limits. As an example, one fairly obvious parameter is temperature. Cells can literally freeze to death when the watery fluids turn into ice crystals that pierce the delicate cell membranes. They can also overheat and die when chemical reactions speed up (as occurs in a fever) and then begin to change the nature of chemicals (as when the liquid albumen of an uncooked egg turns into the solid white of a boiled egg). Such is the self-regulating nature of living organisms that any deviations from the optimum conditions in the body tend to cause responses that return the system to the optimum. Thus when our body temperature falls we start to shiver. The heat generated by the muscle movements involved in shivering will tend to return body temperature to normal. In the 1930s American physiologist Walter Cannon coined the term **homeostasis** to describe the various physiological systems that serve to restore the normal state, once it has been disturbed. Many biologists prefer to use the term **homeodynamic** because the normal state is not necessarily fixed at one level but may vary depending on the situation. For example, in Book 4 you will see how our body temperature fluctuates in a regular way over a 24-hour cycle.

Homeostasis is an essential biological principle with two important and related aspects.

- Life is only possible provided that certain key variables of the body are maintained within limits.

- Deviations from these optimum conditions in the body tend to cause responses that return the system to the optimum.

The type of response that we examined above (shivering in response to a fall in temperature) is an example of a **negative feedback** response. Negative feedback is the process by which a control mechanism reacts to a change in the output of the system by initiating a restoring action. Negative feedback systems maintain a preset state, so they are stable and an important feature of homeostasis. Although negative feedback is crucial in re-establishing normal conditions when deviations occur, it is not the only homeostatic mechanism involved in the maintenance of the internal environment.

- Think about your own experiences and try to recall some examples of where homeostasis is maintained by your behaviour even though no deviations from normal have yet happened.

- In winter you might put on warm clothes before leaving your centrally heated home. On a hot summer day you might consume a cool drink even before losing significant body water or feeling uncomfortably hot. Visitors to the tropics will often take in extra salt before they travel (we lose a lot of salt in sweat). These are all anticipatory, pre-emptive actions.

Such anticipatory actions as taking salt tablets are, in effect, a process that is termed **feedforward**, to distinguish it from feedback control where the response is to a disturbance that has already occurred.

The above examples of feedforward control are forms of behaviour that we perform in full consciousness of their effects and with this purpose in mind. In fact, there are other, involuntary, feedforward mechanisms which also play an important role in homeostasis. You will learn more about these, particularly in Book 2.

The important variables critical for life that are held within limits are said to be **regulated variables**. The processes that serve such regulation are said to be **controlled processes**. Thus shivering is controlled in the interests of body temperature regulation. Shivering can be at a high or low level or may not occur at all, all in the regulation of temperature (i.e. **thermoregulation**).

Thus there is a biological imperative that regulated variables are held nearly constant irrespective of circumstances. By contrast, there are other variables, such as shivering, involved in these processes that may need to vary considerably, according to circumstances. Although the distinction between regulated and controlled variables is an extremely useful concept to aid our understanding of how the internal environment of the body is maintained, it is not always clear-cut. For example, heart rate (a controlled variable) can only vary *within restricted limits* to subserve the maintenance of oxygen levels in the blood (a regulated variable).

Because all the processes that characterize life can take place in a single cell our study of human biology necessarily requires an understanding of the metabolic processes that occur in cells. First, however, we need to know more about the structure and function of cells.

Summary of Section 2.4

1   Living organisms are self-regulating and direct their own metabolic processes.

2   Homeostasis refers to the ability of physiological systems to hold regulated variables within tightly defined limits. This is a dynamic process of control.

3   A major controlling mechanism is the negative feedback system, but feedforward control may also be used.

2.5 The cell

Figure 2.7 is a schematic diagram of an animal cell. It shows all the key components but as cells are specialized to perform different roles this generalized cell isn't really typical of any to be found in our tissues. The **morphology** (shape) of cells reflects their specific function. For example, the morphology of some neurons resembles a branching tree (Figure 2.8a). This shape increases their surface area and allows them to receive information from many neighbouring cells. In contrast, immune cells circulating in the blood are essentially spherical, allowing them to circulate smoothly in the tubes formed by blood vessels (Figure 2.8b).

Figure 2.7   A schematic diagram of a typical animal cell.

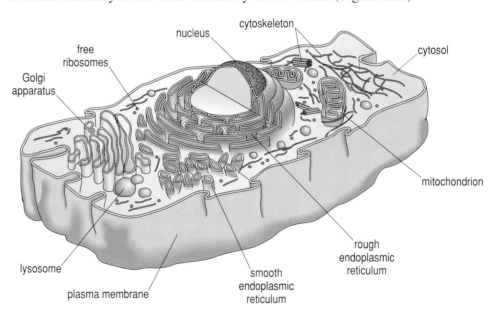

Figure 2.8   Simplified diagrams of (a) a neuron and (b) cells of the immune system.

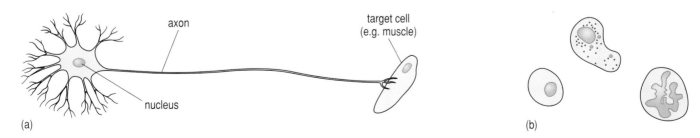

2.5.1 The plasma membrane

Notice that in Figure 2.7 the cell membrane is labelled **plasma membrane**. This is an alternative name for this structure.

● What is the function of the plasma membrane?

○ The plasma membrane is responsible for maintaining the integrity of the cell (Section 1.5).

It keeps the internal fluids and organelles separate from the external environment – the **extracellular** fluids. The membrane is very selective about what it will allow into the cell and also as to what may leave. The consequence of this is that the **intracellular** fluid differs from the extracellular fluid. The concentrations of certain chemicals are different on the two sides of the membrane. In this situation we say that there is a concentration gradient for each of these chemicals across the membrane.

● If there is a concentration gradient what process would you expect to be taking place?

○ When you have a concentration gradient for a chemical that is dissolved in a fluid you expect diffusion to take place (Section 2.3.3).

Figure 2.9 shows the concentration of some major ions on the inside and outside of the part of a neuron known as the **axon** (identify the long tube-like fibre labelled axon in Figure 2.8a). You can see that these ions cannot be diffusing freely across the membrane and in a moment you will find out more about the structure of the membrane and how it controls their passage.

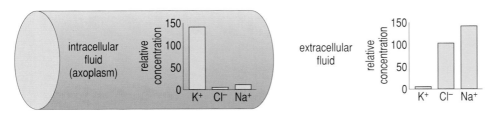

Figure 2.9 The concentration of some major ions on the inside and outside of the axon of a neuron. Note that there are many other ions and molecules present but not shown here.

Because ions are held at different concentrations on either side of the membrane there is a difference in charge across the membrane. One side of the membrane is relatively more positive and the other side is relatively more negative. This difference in charge is called a potential difference and the membrane is said to have a **membrane potential**. All the cells in your body have membrane potentials but in Book 2 you will discover that neurons can *alter* their permeability to specific ions in a quite dramatic fashion. It is this feature that allows neurons to transfer information rapidly over long distances in the body (as electrical signals).

The structure of the plasma membrane is shown in Figure 2.10a (overleaf). It has a homeostatic function in that it is responsible for protecting the finely balanced machinery inside the cell from changes in the extracellular fluid. At the same time the cell's requirements for oxygen and glucose must be met and waste products must be eliminated. So the membrane must selectively permit the entry and

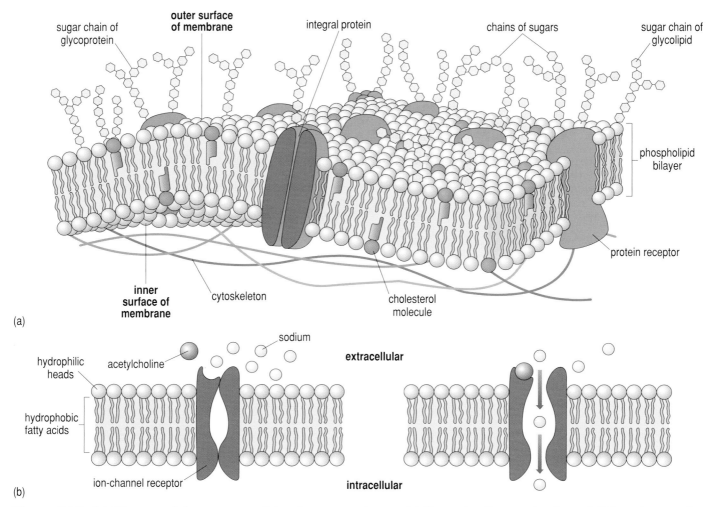

Figure 2.10 (a) Diagram of the structure of the plasma membrane. (b) Example of a protein channel. When the protein receptor is activated by the binding of a specific molecule, e.g. acetylcholine, a change in the structure of the protein follows that allows entry of ions, e.g. sodium, into the cell.

exodus of appropriate molecules and ions. The membrane's selectivity is fine-tuned to the cell's metabolic needs, controlling the direction, amount and timing of the passage of these chemicals.

● Look at Figure 2.10a and identify the regions where molecules could pass through the membrane.

● One possibility is through channels formed by the integral proteins that span the membrane.

Some substances can pass through these channels or pores freely by diffusion (we say that the membrane is *permeable* to these substances). Others are prevented from passing; for example, they might be too large, and so the cell membrane is called a **semipermeable membrane**. In Figure 2.10a the channels look fixed. In reality there are many different types of **membrane protein** and thus many different types of membrane channel and they exhibit considerable fluidity in more than one respect. For example, there is a dynamic turnover of membrane proteins and this is under genetic control. Thus, as gene activity fluctuates, some proteins are broken down but are replaced by similar proteins; others may be removed but not replaced. New proteins may be inserted into the membrane or the density of existing proteins altered.

● Give an example where the changes in the components of the cell membrane give rise to altered properties and ultimately function.

● In the early development of the embryo (at the 16-cell stage), one group of cells have adhesive cell membranes that cause them to recognize one another and cling together as an inner mass that develops into the embryo. In the meantime the outer non-adhesive cells develop to form part of the placenta (Section 1.5).

This change in adhesiveness is a consequence of a change in membrane proteins.

Figure 2.10a also shows a **protein receptor** (mentioned in Section 2.3.2). Protein receptors respond to the presence of certain molecules in the extracellular fluid by inducing a change in the activity of the cell. One such change is the opening of protein channels in the membrane which allows the selective entry of ions into the cell (Figure 2.10b). Sometimes the opening of a channel simply allows ions or molecules to diffuse through the membrane. But there are other membrane proteins ('carrier proteins') that can actively select and carry a substance across the membrane, often working against that substance's concentration gradient. This is known as **active transport** because it requires an input of energy to drive the process.

The major component of the plasma membrane is a double layer (bilayer) of fatty molecules called **phospholipids**. There are many different phospholipids and they are present in different proportions in different membranes.

● In Figure 2.11a (overleaf), there are electrical charges shown on the spherical part of the molecule (head) whilst there are none on the tails. How would you predict that each of these parts of the molecule will behave in water?

● The positively charged head will be attracted to the partial negative charge on the O atoms in water molecules. (Remember water molecules are formed by polar covalent bonding between atoms of oxygen and hydrogen – Section 2.3.3 – overall they are uncharged but they have areas of negativity and areas of positivity, i.e. an unequal distribution of electrons.) The uncharged tails will not interact with water.

Molecules that carry a charge tend to associate with water molecules easily and are said to be **hydrophilic** ('water-loving'). By contrast uncharged and non-polar molecules do not associate with water. They are called **hydrophobic** ('water-hating').

● Fats are uncharged, non-polar compounds. How does fat behave in water?

● Fat does not mix (associate) with water. It forms discrete droplets.

All phospholipids are formed from chemicals called fatty acids and glycerol together with another group of atoms that include a phosphorus (P) atom (Figure 2.11b). The tails of the phospholipids are formed of fatty acid chains and being hydrophobic they cluster away from the water. So with a 'water-loving' head and a 'water-hating' tail it is natural for phospholipids to arrange themselves as a bilayer with heads in contact with water and tails turned away, as shown in Figure 2.10a. Figure 2.11b shows the **structural formula** of a phospholipid molecule. (A structural formula shows how atoms are joined together. The structural formula for water is: H–O–H.) All phospholipid molecules are able to move within their membrane layer, their tails rotating and flexing. This results in the membrane being a fluid structure. However, some form of mechanical support is given to cell membranes by cholesterol, another fatty molecule, but one that is structurally very different to the phospholipids and belongs to a group of chemicals known as **steroids**.

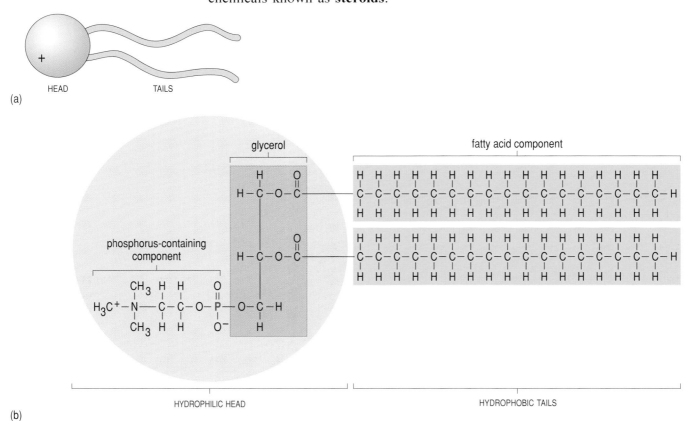

(a)

(b)

Figure 2.11 (a) Diagrammatic representation of a phospholipid molecule. (b) Structural formula of a phospholipid molecule.

The two layers of the membrane are not symmetrically arranged. There are chains of sugars on the outer surface. Some of these form compounds with proteins (**glycoproteins**) and some form compounds with lipids (**glycolipids**). The glycoproteins recognize and receive signalling molecules such as hormones.

● What role do these glycoproteins have in the cell?

◗ They are receptors.

Attached to the inner surface of the membrane are cytoskeletal filaments. Cells have an internal frame, termed the cytoskeleton (Figure 2.10a), which helps the cells to maintain their shape.

2.5.2 Intracellular features

Inside the plasma membrane lie the organelles surrounded by a fluid substance known as the **cytosol**. Each organelle is surrounded by a bilayer membrane, similar to that of the plasma membrane. The most prominent organelle is the nucleus. It is estimated that two metres of DNA is tightly packaged within the nucleus of each cell. DNA molecules are organized into genes (Figure 2.12a) which are functional units that carry the information that passes from one generation to the next. Genes are arranged into single, linear strings of DNA called **chromosomes**, the number of which varies between species. In humans, there are 46 chromosomes: 22 pairs of identical chromosomes plus two sex-specific chromosomes – you either have two X chromosomes, in which case you are female, or an X and a Y chromosome (male) (Figure 2.12b). Gametes only have 22 chromosomes, one of each pair. Sperm have a Y chromosome or an X chromosome, the ovum an X chromosome. The zygote is formed from the fusion of the two gametes and so has 46 chromosomes. It has inherited half of its chromosomes from the mother's ovum and half from the father's sperm.

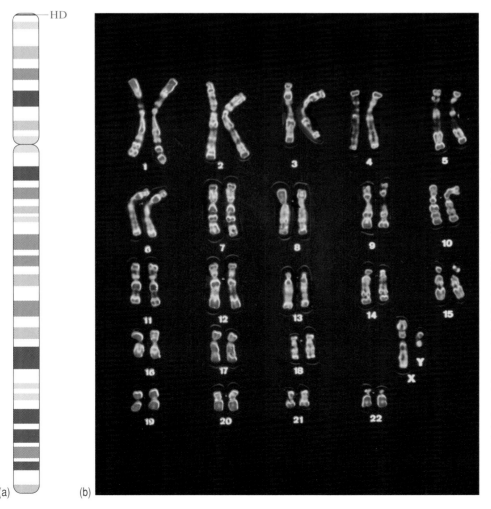

Figure 2.12 (a) Diagram of human chromosome 4. Human chromosome 4 is a linear string of DNA which contains 1631 genes (the darker bands represent areas that can be stained with dyes – they are not individual genes). One example is the Huntingtin gene (HD in red) whose abnormal length is characteristic of patients with Huntington's disease, a disorder characterized by uncontrolled movements and dementia. (b) The chromosomes of a human male, magnified approximately 1000 times. The chromosomes have been stained, photographed and arranged in a conventional manner to show the 22 pairs of identical chromosomes plus the X and Y sex-specific chromosomes.

The oval-shaped structures with zig-zag internal organization in Figure 2.7 are the **mitochondria** (singular: mitochondrion). These are responsible for producing a molecule called **adenosine triphosphate (ATP)** which captures energy from nutrients such as sugars (e.g. glucose) and fats by the process of cellular respiration. ATP can be thought of as an 'energy currency' (like money) which can be made and then spent to get things done. Mitochondria are often described as the 'powerhouses' of the cell. When energy requirements are high they use large quantities of glucose to manufacture ATP and they also produce heat as a by-product.

The network of membranes that forms tubes and sacs is known as the **endoplasmic reticulum (ER)**. It is mainly responsible for the synthesis of many molecules important for cellular life such as proteins and lipids. The ER is divided into two types, according to whether they are associated with **ribosomes** (sites of protein synthesis) or not.

- Smooth ER does not contain ribosomes and is involved in lipid synthesis.

- Rough ER is associated with dense globule-shaped ribosomes. Its role in protein synthesis will be described in the next section.

The proteins synthesized in the rough ER are transported to the **Golgi apparatus**. This structure consists of stacks of flat membrane-like sacs in close proximity to many round 'bags' of membranes of various sizes, termed **vesicles**. Newly synthesized proteins are modified and sorted in the Golgi apparatus through this arrangement of sequential sacs to produce proteins of the correct structure. These fully functional intracellular proteins are ultimately packed into vesicles which are then directed to appropriate places within the cell. In a way, proteins are 'delivered' from the Golgi apparatus to where they are needed within the cell by use of this vesicular system.

Proteins within vesicles can also be exported out of the cell, a process termed **exocytosis** (from the Greek *exo*, outside and *cyt*, cell) (Figure 2.13a). The reverse process by which molecules outside the cell are taken into the cell is termed **endocytosis** (*endo*, inside) (Figure 2.13b). Endocytosis is achieved by engulfing extracellular material into round vesicles formed by invaginations ('dimples') of the plasma membrane. Once inside the cell these vesicles are directed to the Golgi area where their contents, if not required for cellular processes, are broken down by proteins located within small organelles known as **lysosomes**. Lysosomes are also responsible for degrading waste material or unwanted organelles in the cell.

It is now time to turn to the detail of one of the most important of cellular activities: how genes make proteins.

Figure 2.13 (a) The events of exocytosis in which proteins and other intracellular material are secreted from the cell following fusion of a vesicle with a plasma membrane. (b) The sequence of events in endocytosis, by which material is taken into a vesicle formed by invagination of the plasma membrane. The photographs 1–4 relate to the stages numbered on the diagram. The scale bar is given in units of μm (micrometres). 1 μm is a unit of length that is a thousand times smaller than 1 mm (1000 μm = 1 mm).

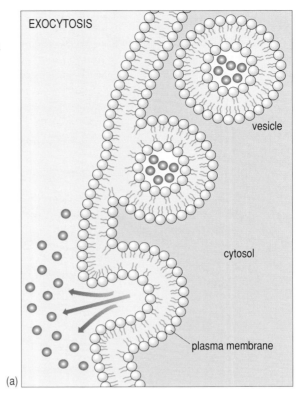

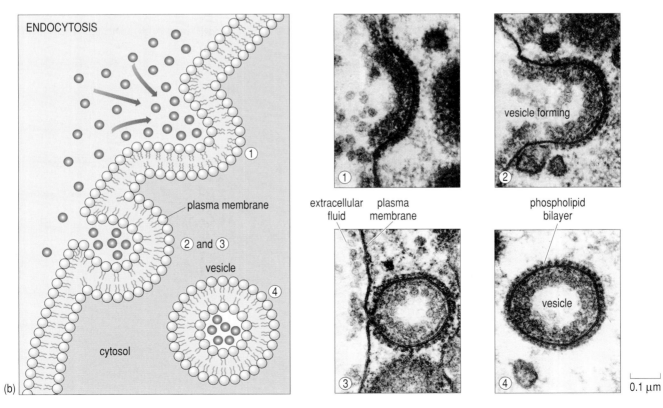

Summary of Section 2.5

1   The cell membrane is a selectively permeable barrier, controlling the cell's internal environment. It is composed mainly of phospholipids, with cholesterol and various proteins; many membrane lipids and proteins have sugar chains attached.

2   The roles of membrane proteins include solute transport, cell–cell recognition and binding of chemicals to receptor sites.

3   The fluid structure of the cell membrane allows it to engulf and ingest material (via endocytosis).

4   Cells contain fluid contents (the cytosol) plus a range of structures (organelles).

5   The cell organelles include the mitochondrion, which carries out cell respiration, and the lysosome, which is involved in intracellular digestion and recycling of materials.

6   The endoplasmic reticulum (ER) is a membrane system within the cell; many of the ribosomes (structures involved in protein synthesis) are attached to the ER.

7   The Golgi apparatus is another intracellular membrane system – it is involved in protein processing and export.

2.6 The structure of DNA

The genetic material comprises several lengths of DNA, each length being formed from two strands of DNA joined together in a characteristic double helix structure (Figure 2.14).

DNA is a macromolecule made up of repeating molecular units called nucleotides. Each nucleotide consists of three components: phosphate, a sugar molecule and a base (Figure 2.15a). The phosphate and the sugar are the same in each nucleotide but the base can differ. There are four different bases in DNA: adenine (A), guanine (G), cytosine (C) and thymine (T).

In each DNA strand the phosphate of one nucleotide is joined to the sugar of the next nucleotide, and so on down the strand. The two strands are held together by bonds between opposite bases, always A to T and C to G (Figure 2.14b, c). The actual order of the four bases in the genetic material of any one species is remarkably stable. The exact sequence of bases in one of the strands (the *template strand*, described below), determines two things.

*   First, it determines the exact sequence of bases in the other strand (A to T, C to G).

*   Second, the exact sequence of bases in the template strand determines the exact sequence of amino acids in the proteins it codes for, and as you have seen (Section 2.3.2), the exact sequence of amino acids in a protein determines whether or not that protein can function by affecting its shape and composition.

It is the precise sequence of bases in the template strands of DNA that is the genetic material and comprises the information that is passed from generation to generation in the egg and sperm cells.

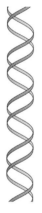

Figure 2.14 Schematic drawing of DNA showing how two strands are linked in a double helix structure.

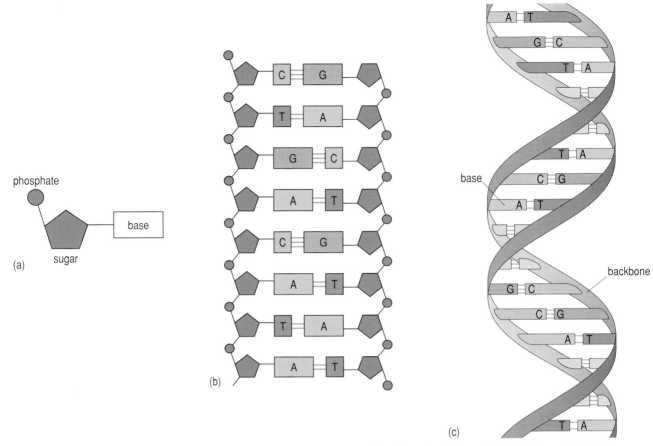

Figure 2.15 (a) A nucleotide composed of a phosphate, a sugar molecule and a base. (b) A portion of a DNA molecule with the helix unwound, showing the complementary base pairs between the two strands held together by base-pairing interactions (shown as orange lines). A = adenine, T = thymine, C = cytosine and G = guanine. (c) Illustration of part of a molecule of DNA showing how the two strands are linked by the bases.

It is an incredible fact that, although the cells in your body are diverse, virtually every one of them carries a complete and exact copy of the genetic material with which you were endowed at conception! A pristine copy of the genetic material in each cell allows the cell to continually break down its current stock of proteins and replace them with new proteins produced from the DNA template. This turnover of proteins is necessary to ensure the current set of proteins is appropriate and functioning. DNA is not subject to any 'turning over' and remains pristine for the life of the cell.

Not all the DNA codes for protein. This is certainly true for the non-template strand, but it is also true of the template strand. Some DNA of the template strand seems to do nothing at all and other bits of DNA act as attachment points for the proteins that control, and the enzymes that undertake, the decoding process.

A section of DNA that codes for a protein is called a **gene**. A gene may be a single continuous section of DNA, but it may not be. All the genes contained within the cells of an organism are called the **genome** or genotype of that individual. As there are many thousands of proteins, and each protein is coded for by a particular gene, it follows that there must be many thousands of genes. These genes are arranged so that there are very many genes in one template strand of DNA. The genes are strung together in a precise order and interspersed with the non-coding sections of DNA, sometimes disparagingly termed junk DNA. Amazingly, around only 1.5% of the human genome codes for proteins. When a cell is actively producing a protein we say the genes involved are being expressed.

2.7 The function of DNA

The amino acids that form proteins are joined together with the help of ribosomes in the cytosol of the cell (Figure 2.7). The mechanism by which the information encoded in the DNA (in the nucleus) is brought together with the ribosomes involves an intermediary molecule. The intermediary molecule is ribonucleic acid (RNA) and it carries the message from the template strand in the nucleus to the ribosomes, hence the name **messenger RNA (mRNA)**.

Unlike DNA, mRNA molecules are not present in the nucleus all the time but are made specifically to order using a short section of DNA as a template. The process of using the template to make a complementary RNA strand begins with a part of the DNA double helix (Figure 2.16a) unwinding and separating its two strands (Figure 2.16b), in response to molecular signals. RNA is made along *one* of these strands, the template strand, by following a very similar pairing procedure to that used between the two strands of the DNA molecule (Figure 2.16c).

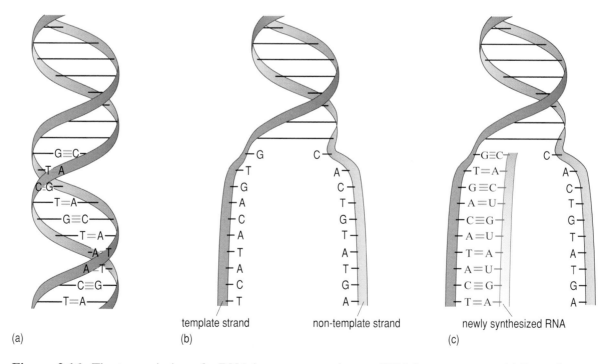

(a) (b) template strand non-template strand (c) newly synthesized RNA

Figure 2.16 The transcription of a DNA base sequence into an RNA base sequence. (a) Part of a DNA double helix showing a few base pairs. (b) The same DNA double helix but unwound to reveal two sets of bases. (c) The unwound DNA molecule showing the synthesis of a molecule of RNA on the template strand. (*Note:* In RNA the pairing is the same except thymine is replaced with another base called uracil.)

A protein, RNA polymerase, is responsible for matching RNA bases to DNA bases and joining the RNA bases together. RNA polymerase attaches to the start sequence of the exposed DNA and using the nucleotide bases present in the cytosol builds a chain of bases complementary to the DNA bases on the template strand; this process of synthesizing RNA on a DNA template is called **transcription**. Note that the non-template strand of DNA has the same sequence of bases as the RNA product, albeit with thymine replacing uracil. When the RNA polymerase reaches the stop sequence of the exposed DNA, a particular sequence of three bases, transcription is complete. The single-stranded RNA molecule detaches from the DNA template strand, allowing the DNA to rewind itself.

The newly synthesized mRNA molecule is transported out of the nucleus, across the nuclear envelope (membrane) with the aid of specialized and specific transporter proteins. (This is an example of the way that membranes can control which substances cross them.) Once in the cytosol, ribosomes become attached to the mRNA and the process of **translation** into a protein begins (Figure 2.17).

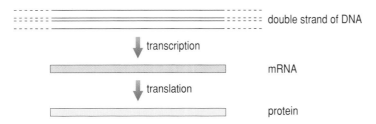

Figure 2.17 Information flow from DNA to RNA to protein.

The ribosomes match the sequence of bases in the RNA to the appropriate amino acids in the cytosol, join those amino acids together and produce a protein.

● Will one base specify one amino acid?

● No, as there are only four different bases but 20 different amino acids.

A two-base code would only provide $4 \times 4 = 16$ permutations; a three-base genetic code provides $4 \times 4 \times 4 = 64$ permutations. By using a three-base code each amino acid can be uniquely coded. A three-base sequence that is 'read' by the ribosomes is called a *codon* and a given codon corresponds to a particular amino acid. There are more codons available than there are amino acids and most amino acids are coded for by several different codons.

It was mentioned earlier that a section of DNA that codes for a protein is a gene. However, the word 'gene' is actually a collective term, like the terms socks and rose – there are a number of different types of socks and a number of varieties of rose. Let us take the case of the enzyme that breaks down alcohol, alcohol dehydrogenase. Everyone has genes that code for this protein but they are not all exactly the same. Different varieties produce enzymes that catalyse at different rates, or produce the enzyme more slowly so that there is less available to break down the alcohol.

● What effect would be noticed if an individual produced below normal levels of alcohol dehydrogenase or a variety of the enzyme that was slow to break down alcohol?

● That individual would become more readily intoxicated and would also remain intoxicated for longer.

You may have noticed that individuals do vary in their response to alcohol. Everyone carries genes that code for production of alcohol dehydrogenase but different people carry different varieties of these genes. Each variety of a gene is called an **allele.** So, different people may carry different alleles for alcohol dehydrogenase.

At some point after the mRNA has been translated (and there may have been several ribosomes working on it at the same time so many copies of the protein could have been made), production ceases and the mRNA is released from the ribosome and broken down to its component bases ready to be recycled. The synthesis and degradation of mRNA means that there is a continuous *turnover* of mRNA in response to the demands of the cell and the signals it is receiving.

Summary of Sections 2.6 and 2.7

1   A key metabolic process is the turnover of proteins.

2   The assembly of proteins requires enzymes, ribosomes and mRNA, made from a DNA template.

3   The genetic material DNA is contained within the nucleus.

4   A section of one DNA strand is copied by a process called transcription to yield mRNA which is transported out of the nucleus and into the cytosol.

5   In the cytosol, mRNA becomes attached to ribosomes where its sequence of bases is translated into a sequence of amino acids to produce the gene product, a protein.

6   After translation, the mRNA is released from the ribosome and is broken down into its constituent bases.

2.8 Cells into tissues

Our discussion so far has focused on the internal workings of a 'generalized', isolated cell. We now move on to look at cells that have become specialized and work together to perform a particular function. All cells have certain characteristics in common and these have been the subject for much of this chapter. They all have a nucleus (though some – red blood cells – lose it as they mature), a cell membrane and cell organelles. The different groupings of cells can be classified according to structure and function (Table 2.1). A group of cells performing the same function is called a tissue. Figure 2.18 shows a sample of different human tissues as seen under light microscopy.

Cells of specific types are said to be differentiated. As you already know every cell of the body has the same set of genes on the chromosomes in the nucleus but

Table 2.1   Cells classified by function. (Note that cells can have more than one function and therefore be classified into more than one group, e.g. some cells of the immune system are found in the blood and often referred to as white blood cells, some support cells are also contractile, and hormone-producing cells can be classified as epithelial.)

Cell group	Examples	Functions	Special features
epithelial cells	lining of digestive tract and blood vessels, outer layer of skin	as barrier, absorption, secretion	tightly bound together by cell junctions
support cells	fibrous support tissue, cartilage, bone	organize and maintain body structure	produce and interact with extracellular material
cells of adipose tissue (fat tissue)	under skin, around organs	energy store	contain very little cytosol most of cell volume is fat
contractile (muscle) cells	skeletal muscle, heart muscle, smooth muscle	movement	contain protein filaments which mediate contraction
nerve cells (neurons)	brain and spinal cord	direct cell communication	communicate with each other and with other cell types by releasing chemical messengers (fast-acting communication)
gametes (sex cells)	eggs, sperm	reproduction	have half the normal chromosome number
blood cells	circulating red and white cells	oxygen transport, defence	haemoglobin in red cells binds oxygen, white cells recognize and destroy potentially damaging material (e.g. bacteria)
cells of immune system	lymphoid tissues (lymph nodes and spleen)	defence	recognize and destroy potentially damaging material (e.g. bacteria)
hormone-producing cells	thyroid and adrenal glands, pancreas	indirect cell communication (via bloodstream)	secrete chemical messengers into blood (slow, long-lasting communication)

the expression of some genes is tissue-specific. This differential gene expression gives rise to the wide range of different cell types, some of which are shown in Figure 2.18 (overleaf). Such differential expression of particular genes may also be time-dependent, with different genes expressed at different stages of the cell's and the individual's life cycle.

All the cells in a particular tissue function together to perform a specialized function, e.g. **connective tissue** (see Figure 1.8) which, as the name suggests, is the packaging tissue filling up the space around the body's internal structures and **epithelial** (covering) **tissue (epithelium)** which lines cavities (e.g. Figure 2.18a) and covers various structures – including, of course, the whole body, as the outermost layer of the skin.

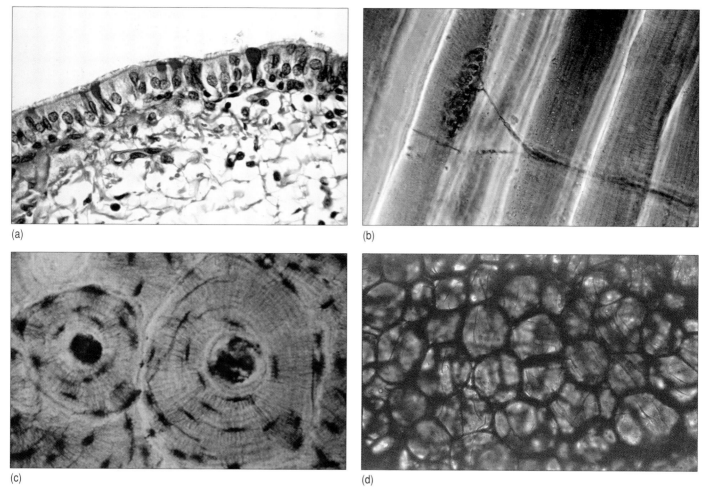

(a)

(b)

(c)

(d)

Figure 2.18 Photomicrographs of some human tissues: (a) epithelium; (b) skeletal muscle with nerve; (c) bone; (d) fat cells or adipose tissue.

Cells of many tissues are held together by a variety of cell junctions which also allow cells to communicate with each other (Figure 2.19). *Tight junctions* connect neighbouring cells together tightly enough to form a fluid-tight seal. Epithelial cells are often joined together by tight junctions and so can act as a barrier to fluid loss. Cells in tissues that are subject to friction and stretching such as the outer layers of the skin, muscle tissue in the heart, the neck of the womb and the epithelial lining of the digestive tract, are commonly joined by different types of *anchoring junctions*. Anchoring junctions use the cell's cytoskeleton (Figure 2.10a) to join cells to one another or to extracellular material (material outside of the cell). A third type of junction is a *gap junction* where adjacent cell membranes come extremely close to each other but do not actually touch. Proteins called *connexins* span the gap, forming fluid-filled channels through which small molecules can pass directly from the cytosol of one cell into the cytosol of a neighbouring cell. Cells that are cancerous do not have gap junctions and so do not communicate well with the cells around them, growing and reproducing in an uncontrolled and uncoordinated way.

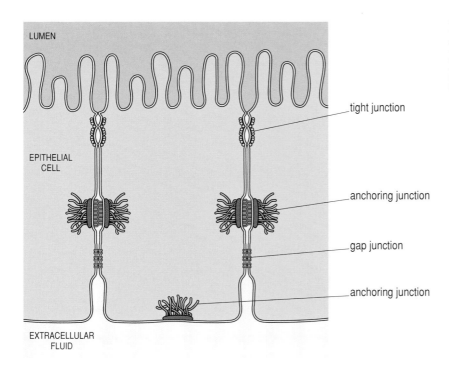

Figure 2.19 Schematic drawing of the different types of junctions between cells. Epithelial cells of the intestine (shown here) possess all these types of junction. Other cell types may only have some types of junction.

Summary of Section 2.8

1   Tissues are groups of differentiated cells performing the same function (e.g. epithelial tissue and connective tissues).

2   The differences between tissues are due to differential gene expression; this can be time-dependent as well as tissue-dependent.

3   Cells in tissues are held together by various types of cell junctions.

2.9 Tissues in action

2.9.1 The healing process

We now focus our attention on a particular and very familiar collection of tissues, the skin, and its response to injury, i.e. the healing process. As you will see, this necessarily requires the production of new cells, an activity that is central to the net growth and repair of all tissues. We shall therefore look in some detail at the process of cell division that leads to the production of new cells.

Healing is by no means limited to the special emergency measures which the body calls upon to restore order to tissues after damage from, say, a skin wound, a sprained ankle, or a broken bone. Healing means 'to restore' or 'to make whole', a process which goes on in organisms all the time. Organisms maintain their structure and form rather as a fountain does: there is a continuous flow of material through the form so that its stability to disturbances comes from a highly dynamic nature, not from static forces such as those that maintain the stable form of, say, a chair or a car. Even our bones are dynamic; if they were not, fractures wouldn't heal. What we see happening in tissues after wounding is just an amplified version of the tissue recycling or turnover which is taking place all the time in the body. (As you know, there is constant turnover at the subcellular level also, with organelles and other cell components being broken down and resynthesized all the time.) In this part of the chapter the objective is to take a look at various aspects of the healing process by examining in detail the structure of the skin and how this structure is restored after wounding. This will take us through the different levels of organization of the body – organs, tissues, cells, and molecules – leading to an understanding of how each of these levels contributes to the integrity of the whole. An essential insight that will emerge is that it is not just what cells and tissues are made of, but more importantly, it is the *dynamic relationships* between the various components that hold the key to living order.

2.9.2 Structure of the skin

The outermost layer of the skin is epithelium. As mentioned in Section 2.8, epithelium forms the surface layer of nearly all the organs of the body, both inside and out. The skin has some important characteristics with which we are familiar. It has a tough surface, is elastic and pliable, hurts when pinched or cut, and has remarkable healing properties, as required of a barrier that separates the body from its physical, chemical and biological environment. When a section of skin is examined under a microscope that magnifies about 100 times, it has the structure shown in Figure 2.20. Starting at the surface (top) and working down, you see several layers and types of cell that are divided into **epidermis** (the epithelial tissue) and **dermis**. These two layers are separated by an undulating single layer of cells shown as little units with dots in the middle, which are the cell nuclei. The highly corrugated structure of the junction between the epidermis and the dermis results in a very strong union that resists shearing forces that might otherwise separate the layers as the skin rubs against objects.

Look at the distribution of the different components in Figure 2.20 – hairs, blood vessels, nerves, muscle – and then try the following questions.

● If a scratch removes only the upper layers of the epidermis, will it bleed?

○ No. The blood vessels are confined to the dermis, so a cut needs to go through the epidermis before bleeding occurs.

● Since the nerves do not extend to the epidermis, why do we feel the light touch of a feather on our skin?

○ We feel it through the hairs, which when moved can activate the associated nerves.

● Do you have any areas of skin that are insensitive to touch? Has this area of skin always been insensitive? If not, why do you think it has lost sensitivity?

○ If you have had a fairly deep wound that removed both epidermis and dermis, including the hairs, then the patch of healed skin can be without hairs or nerve fibres because these fail to regenerate, so the patch will be insensitive. Also, heavily calloused regions of the skin, for example on your feet, become insensitive because the epidermis becomes so thick that a light touch fails to activate any nerves in the dermis.

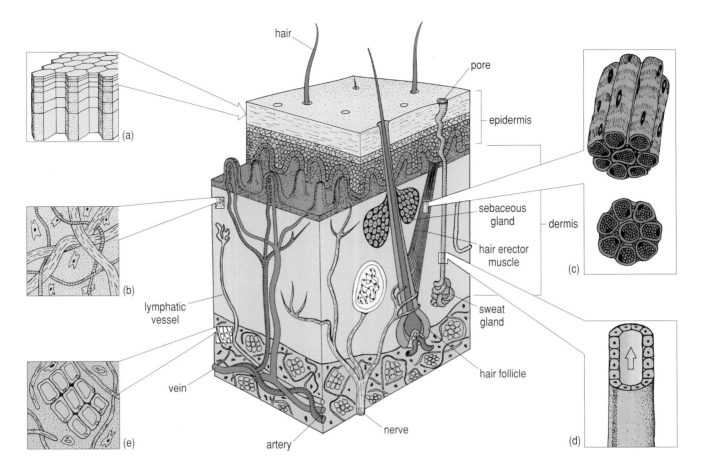

Figure 2.20 Structure of the skin, showing the various types of cells and tissues: (a) epithelial cells in epidermis; (b) connective tissue; (c) muscle; (d) epithelial cells lining the duct (tube) which carries sweat to the surface of the skin. Also shown are (e) adipose tissue just beneath the dermis; this tissue acts as an energy reservoir.

The epidermis has some distinctive features that illustrate the principle that the body is continuously engaged in the healing process to maintain its structure. Inset (a) of Figure 2.20 is a diagrammatic view of the way epidermal cells are organized into hexagonal columns known as epidermal proliferative units (EPUs) – but note that these are not actually visible as discrete units. The structure of a single EPU is shown in Figure 2.21 (overleaf). There are several layers, described as basal, spinous, granular and cornified. Cells in the basal layer are attached to a non-cellular structure, the *basement membrane* (which they produce and maintain), lying just above the dermis. These cells grow and divide, as shown by the cells on the right where the two sets of chromosomes are separating to the two newly formed cells, a stage in the process of cell division (see Section 2.9.3 below). Cells leave the basement membrane to become part of the spinous layer, where they flatten and spread, the nuclei also changing shape. At the same time, these cells begin to produce the protein keratin, which gives the cell mechanical resistance and impermeability. The cells are all attached together by tight junctions (see Section 2.8). Although these junctions are broken down and reformed as the cells move relative to one another, they are very important in maintaining the structural integrity of the epidermis.

Cells in the different layers are distinguished from one another mainly by their content of keratin, which increases towards the surface, as well as by their shape. At the top, in the cornified layer, the cells have become thin desiccated plates filled with keratin and joined together at their edges by very strong tight junctions. They have lost their nuclei and so die, getting sloughed off the surface of the skin as the body goes about its business of interacting with the world. Much of the dust in your house comes from these scales of keratinized skin; most of the rest of it is hair, which is also made of keratin.

Figure 2.21 Section through an epidermal proliferative unit (EPU), showing the layered structure. Cells in the basal layer, attached to the basement membrane, grow and divide. Cells are displaced from the basement membrane and move into the spinous layer, where they flatten and differentiate, producing keratin. The cells (called keratinocytes) are pushed upwards from layer to layer, flattening progressively and producing more keratin until they lose their nuclei and become the hardened scales of the cornified layer.

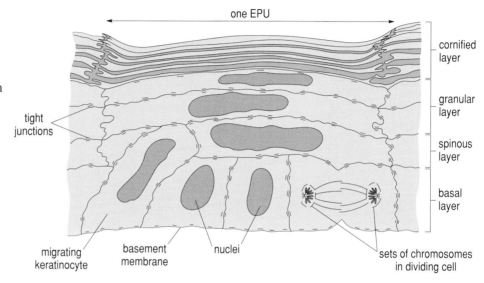

2.9.3 Cell division

The process at the foundation of most tissue maintenance is cell growth and division, whereby one cell gives rise to two. The cells of some tissues turnover very rapidly, for example, the cells lining the gut; others are much slower, for example, heart muscle cells. Cells lost through wear and tear are continuously replaced, normally at a rate that just balances loss. Otherwise, the result would be excessive cell production, leading to a tumour; or deficiency, resulting in tissue wasting. In the epidermis, this actively dividing population is the basal layer. The following account describes cell division with particular reference to the epidermis, but bear in mind that the same sequence of events occurs in *all* the dividing cells of the body.

The cells of the basal layer grow, and at a certain stage of growth the DNA of the chromosomes starts to replicate, i.e. makes a new copy of itself, in preparation for cell division. This DNA **replication** process occurs in the nucleus and takes several hours. First the DNA double helix begins to unwind and split down the middle. Each strand serves as a template for the synthesis of another, complementary strand. Thus two new DNA double helices are formed, each having one strand from the 'old' original DNA double helix and one newly synthesized strand. DNA synthesis begins when a cell receives a signal to reproduce. The important outcome of replication is that the sequence of bases in DNA is faithfully copied from one molecule to the next. This type of nuclear division is called **mitosis**.

Once a basal cell has duplicated its chromosomes, it is well on its way to making two cells, each of which will get a complete set of chromosomes. The sequence of events resulting in the partitioning of the duplicated chromosomes into two nuclei is shown schematically in Figure 2.22 (for simplicity, only four of the 46 chromosomes are shown here). The duplicated chromosomes, at this stage still joined together, first condense into compact structures within the nucleus (Figure 2.22a). (They are now visible under light microscopy.) The nuclear envelope (membrane) then disintegrates and the chromosomes gather at the centre of the cell (Figure 2.22b). A special protein (called the mitotic apparatus), is involved in separating one copy of each chromosome from its duplicate and moving them to opposite poles (ends) of the cell (Figure 2.22c–d). A new nuclear envelope is formed around each of the sets of chromosomes and the cell then divides (Figure 2.22e) into two. Cell division is now complete – one cell has become two, each with a chromosome content identical to that of the original cell.

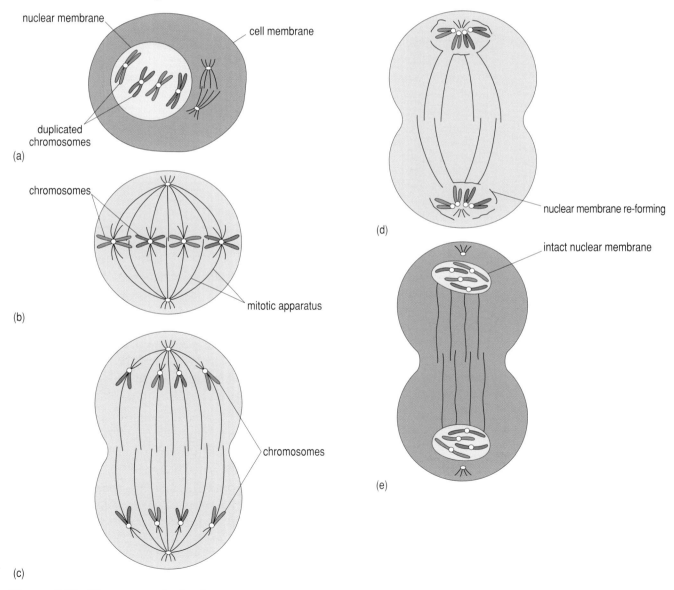

Figure 2.22 The stages of mitosis.

The whole process, from the growth of a newly formed cell through DNA replication and chromosome duplication to the formation of two cells, is called the **cell cycle**. Of course, all the other constituents of the cell described earlier also increase in quantity during the growth phase, so that both new cells have a complete allocation of the materials and structures that make up a living cell. Attention is focused on the chromosomes and the genetic material in this process because of the importance of an equal partitioning of genes to both progeny cells in order that they retain the capacity to grow and to differentiate normally. However, it is important to realize that the total organization of the cell is required for this to occur. What reproduces is the whole cell and this has to be understood in terms of the dynamic interactions of *all* its constituents. This integrated system is more than the sum of its constituent parts, none of which would be able to perform as they do without the presence of the other constituents and their organized interactions. Also, to understand why a cell in a tissue such as the epidermis carries on growing and dividing rather than differentiating into a specialized cell such as an epidermal keratinocyte, we need to take account of its environment, e.g. the location of the basal cell layer in the tissue and the properties of the basement membrane, its position relative to the nutrients that come to it from the blood vessels in the underlying dermis and in relation to differentiating cells above it. These provide conditions and signals that influence cell behaviour in the basal layer, determining how rapidly cells grow and divide, conditions that can be disrupted.

2.9.4 The dermis

Now look back at the structure of the dermis in Figure 2.20. We have already noted the presence of nerves and blood vessels in this tissue and their absence in the epidermis.

● What strikes you as a sharp contrast between the cellular organization of the dermis and that of the epidermis?

◐ There are fewer cells and much larger amounts of connective tissue in the dermis than in the epidermis.

Inset (b) of Figure 2.20 gives a schematic view of the structure of the loose connective tissue of the dermis, which has the appearance of a disorganized tangle of fibres with cells interspersed among them. The thicker threads are fibres of the structural protein **collagen** which have great mechanical strength and elasticity. These fibres form bundles that run in characteristic directions in different parts of the body. You can determine their direction by pinching your skin together and finding out which way it folds most easily into fine wrinkles. After a certain age, no pinching is necessary; the wrinkles are just there. This is because the elasticity of collagen and other fibres gradually decreases with age.

The natural folds of the skin are known as cleavage lines, and they are important to a surgeon: an incision that separates parallel bundles of collagen fibres without rupturing them heals with a fine line, whereas an incision severing and disrupting them produces a broad scar.

● Which way do the collagen fibres run on your torso?

◐ Around it, i.e. transversely.

● So which is the best direction for an incision to remove an appendix?

● A transverse incision.

Within the connective tissue of the dermis are located cells of different type and the various structures such as sweat glands, hairs with associated muscles and sebaceous (oil-producing) glands, vascular tissue (fluid-conducting vessels – arteries, veins, lymphatics) and nerves. The sweat glands secrete sweat onto the surface of the skin, getting rid of some of the body's wastes and at the same time keeping the skin cool. The greasy substance secreted by the sebaceous glands lubricates the skin, keeping it supple and preventing it from drying out. As in the epidermis, the structures of the dermis are dynamically maintained: hairs grow, muscle cells get damaged and are replaced, vascular tissues rupture and are repaired, and collagen gets remodelled in response to the stresses and strains on the skin.

As you can see in Figure 2.20, inset (b), there is more to connective tissue than just collagen bundles. Thinner fibres are entangled with the collagen. These are elastic fibres, largely made up of the protein elastin, which increase the strength of connective tissue. Also present are many types of non-fibrous protein that make up the material between cells and fibres – known as the **extracellular matrix** (ECM). Cells called **fibroblasts** ('fibre cells') move about in the dermal matrix, producing collagen and other constituents of the ECM, which they are continuously remodelling, thereby maintaining a distinctive chemical and structural environment which itself acts on the cells, keeping them in a particular state. When this is disturbed, as we consider next in relation to wounding, the changed environment of the cells stimulates them to act in ways that naturally restores the previous state of dynamic order, which is described as a *steady state* (a balanced condition maintained by continuous restoration of components which are always wearing out and being replaced). This process of maintaining a constant condition by a dynamic balance between opposing forces is another example of homeostasis.

Summary of Section 2.9

1   Healing is an expression of the normal maintenance activities of the body, based on a balance between production and destruction of components.

2   The epidermis is maintained by a dynamic balance involving cell division, cell movement and cell differentiation, the production of extracellular materials and cell death. These processes are spatially organized in epidermal proliferative units, with dividing cells in the basal (bottom) layer and progressively differentiated, keratinized cells in layers up to the surface, where dead cells are removed through wear and tear.

3   Cell division involves chromosome replication and their equal partitioning to the two new cells (mitosis) as well as duplication and partitioning of all other cell constituents, with the result that both progeny cells inherit the entire dynamic organization characteristic of the living state.

4   The dermis is loosely packed connective tissue containing collagen and elastin fibres within an extracellular matrix (ECM) produced and maintained by fibroblasts. Within the dermis are sweat glands, hairs with associated muscle fibres and sebaceous glands, vascular tissue and nerves.

2.10 Wound healing

2.10.1 Tissue damage and pain

The first response to a skin wound is the rapid reflex action that gets the body away from the cause of the damage; the experience that follows quickly is that of pain.

The next stage of the wound response is a temporary recovery of integrity by the processes of blood clotting to cover the exposed area. If the wound involves considerable blood loss (**haemorrhage**) that is not quickly staunched, then mechanisms within the body that rapidly restore blood pressure and blood volume are brought into play, so that the heart continues to function normally (see also Book 3, Chapter 2). These wound-response mechanisms depend upon regulatory processes operating over the body as a whole, not just local ones occurring in the skin. Depending on the severity of the wound, different levels of the body's regulatory activities are brought into operation but here the focus is on the healing processes within the skin itself.

2.10.2 Provisional recovery: inflammation and clean-up

As soon as blood vessels are damaged and blood is released into the wound area, the blood-clotting mechanism is triggered. A protein in the blood plasma (the liquid part of the blood) changes from a soluble form known as fibrinogen to insoluble fibres of fibrin that become tangled together with blood cells and form a dense mat, a fibrin clot. This is a provisional extracellular matrix that is not unlike that of connective tissue with its tangled fibres, but it is made of different proteins and is much denser. As it dries out, this clot forms a scab. In the neighbourhood of the wound, blood vessels **dilate** (increase in diameter) in response to other substances released from disrupted cells, notably a compound called histamine. The dilation makes the vessels leaky so that more blood escapes into the wound region and contributes to clot formation. The dilated vessels can also carry an increased volume of blood to the wound region.

● What are the external signs of this increased blood flow to the wound area?

● Redness and swelling (inflammation).

This is the typical **inflammatory response**: swelling, redness and also tenderness (see also Book 3, Chapter 4). Blood cells get trapped within the fibrin network, particularly the so-called inflammatory cells (white cells). These cells play important roles in healing, by digesting dead cells and tissue remnants and by combating bacterial infection. They do this by engulfing cell fragments and bacteria and then digesting them. This is a particular form of endocytosis called **phagocytosis** (Figure 2.23). White cells also carry out this mopping-up operation within the blood itself, ingesting and digesting damaged and dying blood cells, so that they are continuously involved in this tidying-up process. (And of course, when they die their fragments are ingested by other white cells in the blood.)

cell membrane   dividing bacterium

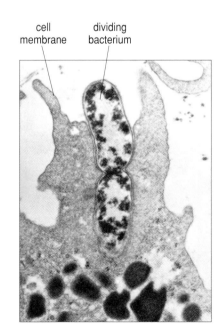

Figure 2.23 A white cell performing phagocytosis. Here, the material being ingested is a bacterium in the process of dividing into two.

2.10.3 Regeneration and repair

As the fibrin clot forms and dries, producing the temporary protective cover of the scab in a few hours, other processes are initiated that bring about tissue regeneration. Blood cells of a particular type, called platelets, release a protein known as platelet-derived growth factor (PDGF), which stimulates cell division in epidermal and dermal cells, and in the white cells involved in clearing up cell debris and engulfing bacteria. In the dermis, the fibroblasts are also stimulated to divide and become more active. They migrate into the wound area, guided by the fibrin network, and differentiate into both collagen-synthesizing cells and cells containing filaments of actin, a protein that gives these cells contractile properties like those of muscle. These contractile cells form in a ring around the wound margin, connecting to one another and to the fibrous components of the extracellular matrix. Their active contraction draws the regenerating dermal tissue inwards over the wound, a process known as **wound contraction**. The fibroblasts produce new collagen and other materials that are laid down as the margin of the wound closes, producing a new extracellular matrix for the regenerating dermis.

In response to PDGF, epidermal cells also become more mobile, migrating over the surface of the closing dermal ring. They secrete materials that become the extracellular matrix of the epidermis, which itself facilitates and guides cell migration. A mere 48 hours after wounding, the surface of the wound may already be covered by a thin layer of epithelial cells. For the next week or so, this grows into the multilayered epithelium of normal skin.

The healing tissue is particularly vulnerable to damage during this phase. The regenerating epithelium is initially a thin layer unable to offer any protection against environmental forces. The same is true of regenerating connective tissue, which does not yet have sufficient strength or elasticity and also contains numerous small, thin-walled blood vessels. At this stage a wound may reopen or bleed as a result of traumas that would be insignificant in normal circumstances. Such damage may delay the healing process or even prevent full recovery if it recurs frequently.

Within the dermis, hair follicles, sebaceous glands, and sweat glands can also regenerate if the wound is not so deep that all remnants of these organs are removed. However, after severe wounding these may not regenerate so that the scar tissue lacks these normal skin components. The new connective tissue has a dense network of blood vessels. This is known as granulation tissue because to the naked eye it has the grainy appearance characteristic of a healing wound (due to the many tiny, newly formed blood vessels within it). The wound is now closed, but the new tissue is still different in many ways from normal skin.

2.10.4 Restitution: remodelling and transformation

The last phase of wound healing involves a process of restitution – the reorganization and remodelling that produces a tissue which is as close as the regenerative process can get to the original structure and properties of the skin. Within the granulation tissue of a wound, the remodelling process begins with the disappearance of many of the (now superfluous) small blood vessels by contraction and closure. Some of the vessels remain to serve the new tissue, those that deliver blood developing a strong, muscular wall and becoming little arteries (**arterioles**) while the veins (which return blood to the heart) retain a thinner, softer wall.

● What do you think the skin looks like at this stage of healing?

● The closing of blood vessels is visible to the eye as a gradual fading of the initially dark purple surface of the wound and the restoration of normal skin colour.

The extracellular matrix of the newly formed dermis has a rather higgledy-piggledy arrangement of collagen fibres, which were laid down quickly by the migrating fibroblasts as the wound closed. These are remodelled by the cells of the dermis so that the fibres become reoriented in the direction of the tension lines of the skin, reforming the cleavage lines described earlier. The elasticity of the tissue is restored by the close packing of the other constituents of the extracellular matrix and the reorganization of the fibres. The epidermis takes on the characteristics of the mature tissue with the reformation of the stacked layers of cells in the hexagonal epidermal proliferative units, though there are often disturbances to the regularity of this arrangement in scar tissue.

The overall result is the restoration of the tough, impermeable, elastic properties of the skin within a period of 2–4 weeks. As stressed earlier, this is achieved by an amplification of processes that continuously maintain the organization of the tissue in its normal state. Some degree of wounding occurs simply as a result of living. For example, exercise may cause minor damage to muscle fibres – hence the need for periods of rest to allow repair. The same is true of disease, which occurs naturally as part of the living process. Health is not, from this point of view, the absence of damage or disease, but the capacity to respond appropriately through a healing process that maintains satisfactory integrity of the body. Healing need not restore the damaged system precisely to its previous state. All that is required is a restoration of function through an adequate structure. In the case of skin, hairs and sweat glands may fail to be regenerated and scar tissue may be less well organized than normal in terms of collagen fibre orientation and the structure of the ECM. Scar tissue is also not as strong and therefore more vulnerable to further damage.

If the skin-remodelling phase does not occur satisfactorily, then the result may be excessive growth and/or disorganization that may lead ultimately to benign or malignant tumours. For example, during wound healing the regenerative phase, initiated by inflammation, may go too far and lead to the formation of superfluous granulation tissue, followed later by fibrosis (primarily, excessive formation of collagen fibres) and contraction which results in malformation, puckering and stiffness, with loss of elasticity. This often happens with burns that have not healed well. Years later, epidermal cancers may occur at these sites. Healing depends upon growth. However, if this is not properly integrated into the other processes of differentiation and remodelling, there is a danger that growth will occur again sooner or later in response to the disorganization, in an attempt to correct it, resulting in cancer (Section 2.13).

Summary of Section 2.10

1   The pain that accompanies a skin wound is an indicator of tissue disorganization.

2   A sequence of events is initiated to restore normal organization after wounding: inflammation and provisional recovery, with scab formation; regeneration and repair, involving cell division, cell migration and extracellular matrix (ECM) formation; and finally, remodelling, resulting in a good approximation to the normal state.

2.11 Nutrition and the healing process

Two of the most important conditions required for rapid and effective healing are adequate nutrition and the absence of infection. In the past, good nutrition and dietary rules were among the most important factors that could be used to facilitate healing. With the advent of antibiotics and powerful, selective synthetic drugs, there has unfortunately been something of a decline in the perceived significance of these basic requirements for the restoration of health, except in the treatment of metabolic diseases (i.e. disorders of cell metabolism), where nutrition is the focus of attention. Patients with serious injuries have an elevated **metabolic rate**, i.e. chemical processes occur more rapidly and they use up large quantities of energy and raw materials.

● What are the raw materials used in metabolism and in what form is energy made available in cells?

● Carbohydrates, lipids and proteins are the raw materials; these are broken down to provide both the 'building blocks' and the energy (as ATP) required for the body's metabolic processes that contribute to growth and repair.

The response to physical trauma is called the **stress reaction**. The regulatory substances released in this response, e.g. platelet-derived growth factor (PDGF) which stimulates growth in epidermal, dermal and blood cells, and stress hormones such as adrenalin and noradrenalin, cause increased rates of use of carbohydrates, lipids and proteins. The body's stores of fat and carbohydrate are mobilized in this heightened metabolic state, which may be accompanied by a rise in body temperature (fever).

● Why does temperature rise in these circumstances?

● The rise in metabolic rate means that the cells are working harder and a by-product is heat.

During the wound-repair phase when the fibres and materials of the extracellular matrix are being laid down rapidly and the connective tissue of the dermis is being restored, there is a greatly increased synthesis of proteins. Any serious protein deficiency in the diet inhibits the formation of granulation tissue, resulting in poor healing of skin wounds. Collagen is particularly rich in certain amino acids (the building blocks of proteins), especially glycine, lysine and proline, so these need to be in plentiful supply, as they are in a well-balanced diet. Other proteins of the extracellular matrix are rich in the amino acids that contain sulfur (methionine and cysteine), adequate amounts of which are therefore also needed in the diet. The formation of collagen fibres, with their elastic and tensile properties, is dependent on a process that requires vitamin C. Thus a deficiency in this vitamin results in poor collagen formation, as well as excessive deposition of other components of the extracellular matrix. The skin is then weak and has a tendency to bleed – hence the characteristic symptoms of severe vitamin C deficiency, scurvy. These consequences of malnutrition also increase susceptibility to infection, which itself delays healing.

In acknowledgement of the consequence of malnutrition, most hospitals employ dieticians to ensure patients are fed properly. So it is with some surprise that even in 2004 there have been cases of hospital patients with symptoms of malnourishment. The Better Hospital Food programme (2004) attempts to eradicate this, putting emphasis on patients being allowed to eat their meals with dignity, for example, without being interrupted by medical staff coming to take samples or to ask questions at meal times.

These basic facts about the importance of good nutrition for wound healing and recovery from illness have been known for many years, but they became firmly established during the 1930s when most of the vitamins were discovered and their therapeutic effects were being recognized. For example, the death rate in children with measles in a London fever hospital was reduced from 8.7% to 3.7% simply by a daily supplement of vitamin A from cod liver oil. The rationing system which ensured an adequate distribution of essential foods and vitamins during and in the period following the Second World War was a spectacular success in practically eliminating malnutrition from the UK.

However, the nutritional status of the population is currently getting worse, though the nature of the problem has now changed. One indicator of nutritional imbalance is obesity, which will be discussed in Chapter 3.

Summary of Section 2.11

1   Successful healing requires good nutrition and the absence of infection.

2   Serious injuries provoke a stress reaction involving the release of hormones that increase metabolic rate throughout the body – often accompanied by fever – and increased growth rates in the damaged tissues.

3   Nutritional deficiencies reduce healing rates and increase susceptibility to infection, which also delays healing.

4   Rationing in the UK during the 1940s and early 1950s improved the nutrition of the population; one current and increasingly serious nutritional problem is that of obesity.

2.12 Stress and healing

The nutritional needs of the body for successful healing tell us about biological factors involved in reconstructing tissues after damage and restoring a functional whole. However, this is only one of the levels that influence the condition of health. Psychological stress and well-being are equally important as factors in healing. A study by an American research team (Kiecolt-Glaser et al., 1995) presented evidence that carers of dependants with Alzheimer's disease recovered from skin wounds significantly more slowly than a **control group** that did not have this responsibility. The investigation involved the study of healthy women in the 47–81-year age group who had been providing care for several years to either a husband or a parent with Alzheimer's disease. They spent an average of 6.7 hours per day in caring activities. Another group (the control group) matched the carers in age, income and social class, but did not have caring responsibilities.

There were 13 carers and 13 in the control group who all agreed to participate in the experiment. This involved making a small wound to the upper arm by a method routinely used to examine skin cells, a procedure called **biopsy**, which produces a very uniform full-thickness wound (i.e. one that removes both epidermal and dermal tissue). The wounds were dressed, then examined at intervals until they were fully healed. The extent of healing was determined by measuring the size of the wound from photographs, and by the response to hydrogen peroxide, an antiseptic that foams when the wound is not fully healed. To avoid observer bias, these measurements were carried out by a person who did not know which were controls and which were carers. Figure 2.24 shows how long it took for a wound to heal completely. The height of the bars gives the percentage of participants whose wounds had healed completely at different times after wounding.

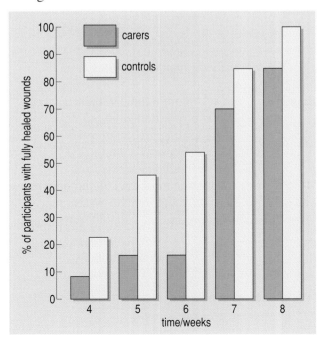

Figure 2.24 Percentage of participants (carers and controls) whose wounds had healed completely, plotted against time after wounding.

● How many people are there in each group and how many people were being studied in total?

● There are 13 people in each group, so 26 people were studied in total.

● How is each individual represented in the Figure?

● The results are represented in a slightly odd way. As there were 13 people in each group it would be possible to have used actual numbers to make a valid comparison. But the experimenters have recorded the percentage of individuals in each group. So each individual is represented as being $1/13 \times 100\% = 7.7\%$ of the group. This is a good way of making comparisons when the groups are not the same size; for example, if one of the participants was unable to continue to take part there would be only 12 in one group and comparing using percentages would be fairer than using actual numbers.

● By the end of the observation period (which Figure 2.24 shows to be 8 weeks) have all participants' wounds fully healed?

● No. The two bars on the right-hand side of the figure show that after 8 weeks there has been 100% recovery in the control group – the white bar – (i.e. all 13 people have fully healed wounds) but the pink bar is showing that just over 80% of the carers are fully healed. That means that there were two individuals whose wounds had still not healed fully.

● If you are a carer will your wounds heal more slowly than those of a person without caring responsibilities?

● Not necessarily. After 4 weeks one carer had a completely healed wound (as represented by the pink bar on the far left of the figure) but only three of the non-carers (the white bar) had completely healed. So there were 10 non-carers who healed more slowly than one of the carers.

This demonstrates a point that was mentioned in Chapter 1 and which you should keep in mind throughout this course; we show tremendous individual variability. It is this variability that makes it difficult to predict how any particular treatment will affect any one individual (see Case Report 2.1 on wound healing) and gives rise to the mistaken 'devil may care' attitude that some people use to justify their maltreatment of their bodies. Who has not heard the argument that: 'My granddad smoked 60 cigarettes a day and lived to 94. Never did him any harm'. Maybe you've even used similar arguments yourself in the past!

● Overall how would you characterize the difference between the two groups shown in Figure 2.24?

● The carers show a delay in healing compared with the controls, though they start to catch up after six weeks.

The investigators also took a blood sample from each individual before the biopsy wound was made. This was used to measure the capacity of the white cells to produce a regulatory protein called interleukin-1, which is important in the formation of the connective tissue matrix and in the migration of fibroblasts. Interleukin-1 levels were found to be significantly reduced in carers compared with controls.

The results of this study, though carried out on a small sample of people, show how psychological stress can affect one of the most basic of the body's repair processes, healing the skin after damage. In Book 4 we return to a fuller discussion of psychological stress and how it can be measured.

● Can you think of another indicator of health that is likely to be affected by psychological stress?

● One of these is vulnerability to infectious disease, which is known to increase in those subjected to stress. (It is also increased by physiological stress, as highly trained athletes are well aware.)

This study points to the significance of what are often called 'states of mind' on the activities of the body, showing that body and mind function as an integrated whole, and that the capacity to heal reflects the condition of the whole person.

Case Report 2.1   Wound healing

Sue is 45 years old and is married with two teenage children. She has a full-time job which she describes as being demanding and stressful. She smokes 20 cigarettes daily and is overweight. She has a longstanding chronic bowel condition but has no other medical problems. She was admitted to a surgical ward for planned major abdominal surgery. She was very anxious about having the surgery and the scar which would result from it, and having to be off work for a long period. After surgery, her wound was closed with clips, these being planned for removal after seven days. Over six million operations were undertaken in the NHS in England and Scotland in 1998/9 (NICE, 2001), and the vast majority of surgical wounds heal without complication, by *primary* intention. This is when in wounds with minimal tissue loss (as in surgical incisions and lacerations), the skin edges are held together by skin closures such as sutures, clips and staples. However, it is estimated that around 21 000 surgical wounds become difficult to heal in England and Wales each year (NICE, 2001). Unfortunately, Sue was one of the unlucky people who developed problems, as five days post-operatively her wound separated (termed 'dehiscence'). It was suspected that this was due to infection as the wound smelt offensive, was inflamed and was producing large amounts of exudate. Sue returned to theatre and an abscess (collection of pus) was drained. It was decided that the wound should be left open to heal by *secondary* intention, which is when wounds are left open, either because the skin edges cannot be brought together due to tissue loss (as in burns or pressure ulcers) or it is inadvisable to close the wound, usually due to infection. Healing by secondary intention is a slower process with healing occurring from the wound base.

Sue was referred to the tissue viability nurses (TVNs), who specialize in wound prevention (in particular, pressure ulcer prevention) and wound management. They applied vacuum-assisted closure (VAC) therapy to the open wound bed. VAC therapy entails localized sub-atmospheric negative pressure being applied via a computerized therapy unit. This removes excess exudate, reduces oedema (swelling), improves circulation, stimulates granulation tissue formation and wound contraction, and reduces bacterial loading. The wound made slow but steady progress in its healing but Sue was very distressed at the condition of her wound and became very depressed about it. She refused to look at the wound and completely lost her appetite. The nurses were concerned that her poor intake of nutrients was impairing her wound healing and she was referred to the dietician. Drinks with added nutrients were encouraged, as well as a nutritious diet, but Sue often felt nauseous and her appetite remained poor. Pain management was also difficult and the acute pain service was involved in helping to achieve a regime which would keep her pain under control.

The TVNs worked hard at building a trusting relationship with Sue, and tried to encourage her to look at the wound so that she could see its progress. Her family were very supportive and encouraging too and eventually Sue agreed to look at the wound and started to accept it. Her mood started to improve and she began to eat better. The nurses noticed that her wound healing started to progress more quickly at this point. Eventually, after nearly two months in hospital, during which she had lost over three stone in weight, Sue was ready for discharge home. Her wound bed was now full of granulating and epithelializing tissue, and there was evidence of wound contraction. The VAC therapy had been discontinued and Sue was now able to dress her own wound. The staff arranged for a district nurse to follow her up in the community for support. Sue had given up smoking in hospital and was determined not to restart. She also planned to reassess her lifestyle and work fewer hours.

Summary of Section 2.12

1   Psychological states such as stress have an influence on healing rates, as indicated by a study of biopsy wound healing in carers of people with Alzheimer's disease.

2   Compared with a control group, the carers had a significantly delayed rate of wound healing and reduced levels of a regulatory protein (interleukin-1) involved in skin regeneration.

2.13 Cancer

In previous sections there have been a number of references to cancer and you may have formed the opinion, correctly, that cancer is a disease of cells. **Cancer** is a diagnostic term for a variety of diseases that can affect any tissue of the body. At the time of writing (2004) it is a major cause of **mortality** (death) in the UK. Many cancers respond to effective treatments though there is considerable variation in the extent to which patients can enjoy good health whilst being treated, so cancer also features prominently in **morbidity** (reported incidence of sickness per 1000 of the population) statistics.

Cancer can be considered to be a genetic disease because it is brought about as a consequence of **mutations** (changes) to specific genes. Mutations can be a result of copying errors occurring during DNA replication. These errors are usually efficiently dealt with by repair enzymes.

● What kind of macromolecule is an enzyme and how is it made?

○ Enzymes are proteins so they are themselves coded for by genes and synthesized on ribosomes.

● What would be the consequence of a mutation in the DNA repair enzyme gene?

○ If there is a mutation in the DNA repair gene the affected cell will not produce normal DNA repair enzymes. Errors would go uncorrected and so mutations would accumulate in cells.

In a normal cell, cell growth and cell division are promoted by **proto-oncogenes**. The activity of proto-oncogenes is kept in check by **tumour-suppressor genes**. Normal growth occurs at a rate that is determined by the balance in activity of these two types of genes as shown in Figure 2.25a.

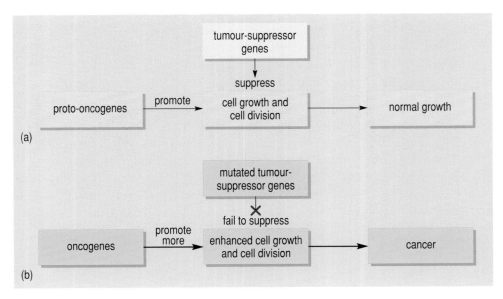

Figure 2.25 Scheme to show the role of genes in the development of cancer. (a) Normal cell growth is controlled by the products of proto-oncogenes and tumour-suppressor genes. (b) Cancer is the result of mutations in both types of gene.

Cancer occurs when proto-oncogenes mutate to become **oncogenes**, which enhance cell growth and division, and tumour-suppressor genes mutate into forms that can no longer oppose the activity of the oncogenes (Figure 2.25b). Carcinogenic (cancer-promoting) substances in the environment increase the likelihood of mutations occurring but cancer is not the result of a single mutation. Rather it results from the accumulation within one cell of a small number of independent mutations that can take place over a long period of time. Figure 2.26 shows how mutations are passed to daughter cells as mutations accumulate randomly over time. Mutations in at least five or six different genes have to accumulate within a cell before it becomes cancerous and this may take place over as long a period as a decade which is why the incidence of cancer increases with age.

Figure 2.26 Over time, a few independently acquired mutations accumulate in one cell and can lead to the development of cancer. For simplicity, only four cell generations are shown, but it takes many more cell generations for a sufficient number of mutations to accumulate in a cell to produce cancer.

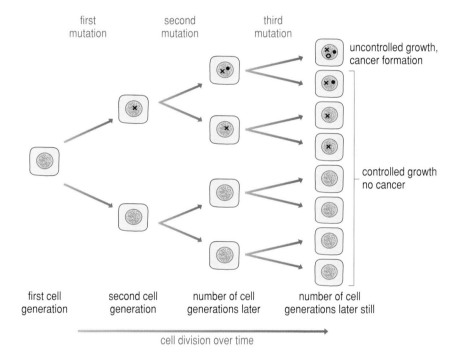

- Cancer only occurs when a particular body cell has acquired a number of mutations. Why then, do you suppose, are some people advised that they may have a genetic predisposition to cancer?

- These people may have inherited a defective allele for *one* of the genes involved in normal cell growth and division. Every cell of their body would have this defective allele but a cancerous growth would only commence when a particular body cell had acquired all the other mutations that are required for the onset of cancer.

In Case Report 2.2 you will notice that the medical team decided that it was unlikely that there was a genetic basis for Mary's breast cancer. In general, currently only 5% of women with breast cancer are thought to have a genetic disposition for the disease.

2.13.1 Carcinogenesis

As an example of disruption of cellular function consider the gene called *RAS*. This gene codes for a protein that is found in cell membranes. The RAS protein responds to signals in the extracellular fluid that tell the cell to prepare to divide.

● What would we call this RAS protein?

● It is a receptor.

The protein changes shape when it receives these signals (Figure 2.27a). But if the *RAS* gene (which is a proto-oncogene) mutates into an oncogene, a defective RAS protein is formed. The defective protein is unable to change shape and is stuck in the shape that it ought only to assume when it gets the signal for the cell to prepare to divide (Figure 2.27b). This means that the chemical machinery that initiates cell division is permanently ready to be switched on.

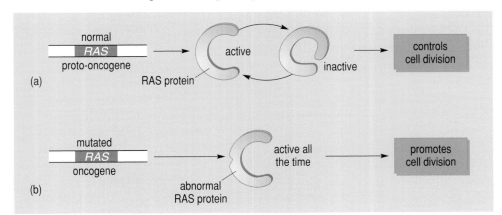

Figure 2.27 The *RAS* gene and the RAS protein: (a) in a normal cell; (b) in a cancer cell. (It is a convention that the gene is written in italics, e.g. *RAS* and the protein in normal script, e.g. RAS.)

As already mentioned a number of mutations to genes and therefore a number of different altered proteins are produced before the cell becomes cancerous and proliferates. But once cells proliferate rapidly they no longer differentiate to form the type of cells typical of the area where they are found.

Carcinogenesis is the development and spread of cancer. It starts as cellular disorganization, at which stage the body's natural defences, such as the immune system, may be able to destroy the offending cells. If this fails, the growth (tumour) will affect the organization of local tissues but may remain, contained within the tissue, for years. However, if the tumour breaks free and gets into the blood or lymphatic system it is likely to initiate growths in other parts of the body. These growths are called secondary cancers or **metastases**.

Cells that are differentiating into a particular type of tissue receive and respond to signals from neighbouring cells. But cancerous cells do not have gap junctions (Section 2.8) and so do not communicate well with the cells around them. Hence they do not respond to the normal inhibitory signals from surrounding tissue. However, they do need supplies of oxygen and nutrients to keep growing and dividing and if this is not met the cells will starve (and be poisoned by their own toxic waste products). A cancerous mass of more than 1 mm in diameter will have cells that are dying off. Such a structure is unlikely to interfere dramatically with surrounding tissue function and fewer than 10% of deaths are caused from tumours such as these. The danger comes from cancer cells that are able to secrete substances that encourage the growth of arterioles into the tumour. These tumours not only grow but the cells more readily break free from one another and travel in the blood system to start the colonization of other body systems.

There are many factors that predispose the development of cancer. The link with smoking is very well known, the effects of diet (the topic of our next chapter) perhaps less generally known, despite the fact that tobacco and diet, between them, account for over 60% of all deaths from cancer.

Case Report 2.2   Breast cancer

Mary is 58 years old and works full-time as a teacher in a special needs school. She lives with her second husband, John, who is a police officer. Her two daughters are both married with children and live some distance away. As part of the NHS breast-screening programme, she was invited to a routine mammogram (breast X-ray). She wasn't concerned about this as she felt fit and healthy and had not detected any lumps. However, a week after the test, she received a letter informing her that she needed further tests, and she was asked to attend the X-ray department at her local hospital for an appointment with the consultant radiologist and breast care nurse. Mary was quite alarmed but tried to be calm about it, hoping it would turn out to be nothing to worry about. John accompanied Mary to the appointment, where a full history was taken, including family history. Mary had no close relatives who had had breast cancer (close relatives are mother, father, siblings, children, aunts, uncles and grandparents). She had a further mammogram, an ultrasound, and a core biopsy, which involved a local anaesthetic and the removal of breast tissue with a needle. Mary also met the breast care nurse, Alison, who explained everything to her, and reassured her that she would be available to support her at each appointment, and that she could contact her between appointments if she wanted to ask questions or discuss concerns.

Mary was told that if the tissue was cancerous, it was very likely that it could be treated successfully as the mammogram had detected it at an early stage. Mary was asked to return for her results two days later. At this appointment she was told that she had breast cancer, but that it appeared to be at an early stage. She was given an appointment to see the surgeon the following week, and some information

leaflets that included telephone numbers to ring for support. Alison spent some time with Mary and John talking through their fears, and explaining what lay ahead for Mary. Mary and John had not yet told their daughters about the diagnosis, and they talked through with Alison how they would approach this. Mary said she'd read that some breast cancers can be genetic, and should her daughters be concerned about this? Alison explained that as Mary had no history of any close relatives having had breast cancer, there was unlikely to be a genetic component. Had there been such a family history, her daughters would have been offered genetic counselling. However, as things stood, Alison explained, they should have no greater risk than any other woman: about a 1 in 9 chance of developing breast cancer throughout a lifetime.

The surgeon recommended that, due to the small size of the lesion, a wide local excision of the lump would be most appropriate, but that lymph nodes must also be removed for examination. Mary was relieved to hear that a mastectomy was not necessary. The surgeon informed her that she would need to see the oncologist (cancer specialist) after her surgery where further treatment for the cancer (radiotherapy, chemotherapy or hormone therapy) could be discussed. Chemotherapy is the administration of anti-cancer (cytotoxic) drugs, which cause cell death by altering DNA and preventing mitosis or by initiating the **apoptotic** (programmed cell death) response. They have a non-discriminatory action on rapidly dividing cells and this leads to range of possible side-effects including alopecia (loss of hair), skin problems, fatigue, gastrointestinal problems, and bone marrow depression. Radiotherapy damages DNA and leads to cell death, particularly at the stage when the cell attempts mitosis. Radiotherapy can be targeted locally, but affects healthy cells in the area too, and side-effects can result. Mary was admitted the following week and the operation was carried out uneventfully. She was able to go home three days afterwards, and was given an appointment to see the surgeon two weeks later. At this appointment Mary was told that examination of tissue removed confirmed that the breast lesion was cancerous, but at an early stage, and that lymph nodes were not involved. She was thus reassured that her outlook was good. The tumour had been found to be oestrogen-receptor (ER) positive, which meant that hormone treatment would be recommended as it significantly reduces risk of recurrence.

Three weeks later, Mary was seen by the oncologist. He explained that as the cancer was at an early stage with no lymph node involvement and as she was post-menopausal, she did not need chemotherapy, but should have a course of radiotherapy. Mary was started on hormone therapy of tamoxifen 20 mg daily, which blocks the effects of oestrogen on cancer cells preventing them from growing. She was told that recommendations, based on best evidence, are that she should stay on this for five years. Her radiotherapy regime was explained, which was to be treatment for several times a week for five weeks. Mary found the radiotherapy very tiring, but remained positive in her outlook. John's colleagues were very helpful in enabling him to arrange his shifts so that he could accompany her for her treatment. Once the radiotherapy was completed Mary was given a follow-up appointment for three months later, and advised that she would need a mammogram a year after her original one. Mary was able to return to work fairly quickly, much relieved that the surgery and radiotherapy were all completed and that her cancer had been found so early.

Summary of Section 2.13

1   Cancer occurs as a consequence of the accumulation of mutations (changes) to specific genes.

2   When cells of a tumour spread they can initiate disorganized growth in other parts of the body.

Questions for Chapter 2

Question 2.1 (LOs 2.1, 2.4)

Figure 2.5 shows human haemoglobin. It is made from four chains of amino acids (i.e. four polypeptide chains). In the sixth position along the globin chain is the negatively charged amino acid called glutamic acid. If there is a mutation that results in valine (a non-polar amino acid) replacing glutamic acid at position 6, the person who carries this mutation has a blood disease called sickle-cell disease syndrome.

Explain how this single substitution of an amino acid in a molecule that is made of 574 amino acids could so dramatically alter the function of the protein.

Question 2.2 (LO 2.2)

An enzyme is found that is required to catalyse a step in the pathway that leads to the production of ATP. However, it is noted that ATP can reversibly bind to the enzyme (i.e. if levels of ATP are high some ATP molecules become attached to the enzyme but they detach from the enzyme when ATP levels drop.) When ATP attaches to the enzyme, the enzyme becomes inactive.

Explain these observations.

Question 2.3 (LO 2.3)

Suggest explanations for the following.

(a) New-born babies have considerable deposits of a particular type of adipose (fat) tissue which appear brownish because of the large numbers of mitochondria present in the cells. New-borns have considerable resistance to low temperatures.

(b) There are epithelial cells lining the intestinal tract that secrete a lubricating mucus (a glycoprotein) and which contain many Golgi sacs and mucus-containing vesicles.

Question 2.4 (LO 2.4)

When epithelial cells in the skin differentiate into keratinocytes the gene for keratin is expressed. Briefly outline the processes involved.

Question 2.5 (LO 2.5)

How does a cell partition complete sets of chromosomes to the two daughter cells that are produced when it divides?

Question 2.6 (LO 2.6)

A friend of yours, who spends many hours every day caring for a member of her family with Alzheimer's disease, has a fall and suffers severe grazing on an arm. You observe that the wound is not healing normally, showing persistent tenderness and redness although it is not infected. What would you assume to be happening, and why? What advice would you give to your friend to improve the healing of her wound?

References

Better Hospital Food programme (2004) [online]. Available at: http://patientexperience.nhsestates.gov.uk/bhf/bhf_content/home/home.asp (Accessed July 2004)

Kiecolt-Glaser, J. K., Marucha, P. T., Malarkey, W. B., Mercado, A. M. and Glaser, R. (1995) Slowing of wound healing by psychological stress, *Lancet*, **346**, 1194–1196.

National Institute for Clinical Excellence (2001) *Guidance on the use of debriding agents and specialist wound care clinics for difficult to heal surgical wounds*. London: NICE.

CHAPTER 3

NUTRITION

Learning Outcomes

After reading this chapter, you should be able to:

3.1 List the six key nutrient groups and explain their role in a healthy diet.

3.2 Explain the importance of a balanced diet in terms of nutrient and energy intake.

3.3 Understand and calculate body mass index (BMI), and use such calculations to predict desirable weight ranges for individuals.

3.4 Describe the structures and roles of proteins, carbohydrates and lipids.

3.5 Give an outline of disorders associated with either deficiencies or excesses of proteins, carbohydrates and lipids in the diet.

3.6 Explain how vitamins and minerals contribute to the body's health.

3.7 Use data from relevant graphs and tables to inform dietary choice.

3.1 Introduction

What is a healthy diet? There are people living all around the world who are healthy but who eat very different diets. The Japanese currently have the longest documented life expectancy of all nationalities and the Okinawans (who come from a small island in the southern archipelago of the Ryukyu islands in Japan) have the longest life expectancy in the world (Cockerham et al., 2000). In 1996 the number of centenarians in Okinawa was 22.14 per 100 000 people, which is more than double the number (approximately 9.5 per 100 000) in England and Wales (Thatcher, 1999). There are a number of factors that may contribute to the longevity of the Okinawans; these include strong family bonds and respect for the elders, living in a warm subtropical climate and healthy dietary habits. The Okinawan diet consists of lots of fresh fruit, vegetables and fish and there is little consumed in the way of convenience foods. There is a very low incidence of obesity in Okinawa that may be associated with the Okinawan philosophy of only eating until they are nearly – about 90% – full. In the western world, obesity is an ever-increasing problem, particularly in the USA and UK.

This chapter will look at the role of **nutrition** (the taking in and assimilation of food by chemical changes) in maintaining good health.

● Is this definition of nutrition holistic or reductionist?

● It is a reductionist definition. It takes a biological perspective.

This is not the only way to define nutrition. A recent textbook on nutrition notes that one possible definition is:

'the study of the relationship between people and their food.'

(Barasi, 2003)

An essential aspect of maintaining the body is the consumption of food. The range of foods that we eat is known as our **diet** and the components of food that are digested, absorbed and used in bodily functions are known as **nutrients**. Nutrients supply the body with both energy and with the components for growth and repair. In this chapter we will examine the various roles of nutrients within the body and look at the effects of nutrient deficiencies or excesses, both of which can lead to adverse health effects.

3.2 A balanced diet

3.2.1 The components of a balanced diet

A balanced diet contains six key nutrient groups that are required in appropriate amounts for health. These groups are outlined below and will be discussed in more detail later in the chapter.

- Proteins are involved in growth, repair and general maintenance of the body.

- Carbohydrates are usually the main energy source for the body.

- Lipids or fats are a rich source of energy, key components of cell membranes and signalling molecules, and as myelin they insulate neurons.

- Vitamins are important in a range of biochemical reactions.

- Minerals are important in maintaining ionic balances and many biochemical reactions.

- Water is crucial to life. Metabolic reactions occur in an aqueous environment and water acts as a solvent for other molecules to dissolve in.

A deficiency of any one type of nutrient can lead to disease, starvation (or dehydration in the case of water) and subsequent death. **Fibre** is a component of food that is not nutritious but is important to include in our diet. Fibre or roughage is non-digestible carbohydrate and it has an important role in aiding the movement of food through the gut.

There is also an absolute requirement for some specific molecules in the diet. This is because, although the body can manufacture most of the molecules it needs, some essential molecules *cannot* be made by the body. These molecules are called **essential nutrients**, and *must* be supplied in the diet, for example lysine and methionine, which are essential amino acids.

Other components of the human diet are not nutrients at all, as they do not perform the functions of producing energy or promoting growth and repair, but are eaten for other purposes. For example, spices and other flavourings help make food more palatable; tea and coffee drinks provide a good source of water and may also contain other valuable substances such as antioxidants (see below).

An adequate diet is essential for health and education plays a key role in providing people with the knowledge of what constitutes a healthy diet, but as is so often the way with science, the information keeps changing. The information about what we should be eating comes from various sources: in the UK a large amount of data was collected and published by COMA, the Committee on Medical Aspects of

Food Policy (1991). This committee has now been disbanded, but its publications still represent a valid source of information about diet. Currently (2004), the Scientific Advisory Committee on Nutrition (SACN) advises the Department of Health and the Food Standards Agency (FSA). The Food Standards Agency produces a guide to choosing a healthy diet, 'The balance of good health', a version of which is illustrated in Figure 3.1. A lack of an adequate supply of any nutrient is known as **malnutrition** and leads to poor health.

● Does Figure 3.1 enable you to identify any nutrient that might be inadequately represented in your diet?

● Figure 3.1 is a representation known as a pie chart. It enables you to see the relative proportions of each of the food categories that are likely to make up your diet. It is a fairly crude instrument and does not allow you to identify any nutrient deficiency.

Figure 3.1 can be useful tool for teaching children about a healthy diet.

● How much fruit and vegetables should you eat?

● Fruit and vegetables should make up over a quarter of your daily intake.

The message in Figure 3.1 is simple and it emphasizes balance rather than focusing on specific nutrients.

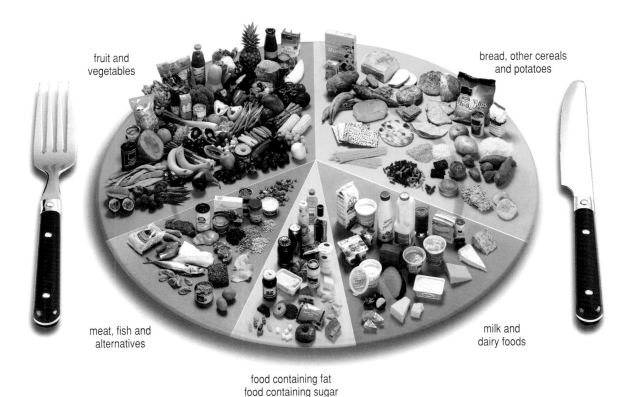

Figure 3.1   'The balance of good health': A guide to choosing a healthy diet.

However, SACN does recommend a range of intake levels for all nutrients and energy for males and females throughout life, known as the **dietary reference values (DRVs)**. Because individuals vary in their exact energy requirements, depending on sex, age, occupation and many other factors, often the **estimated average requirement (EAR)** is given, with the understanding that some individuals need more than this value and others less. EAR values for energy are shown in Table 3.1.

Table 3.1 Estimated average requirements, EAR, for energy throughout the lifespan. Also shown are the extra (+) amounts of energy required during pregnancy and lactation. Values based on COMA data published by the Department of Health in 1991. At the time of writing these are the most recent data available.

Age	EAR/kcal per day	
	Males	Females
0–3 months	545	515
4–6 months	690	645
7–9 months	825	765
10–12 months	920	865
1–3 years	1230	1165
4–6 years	1715	1545
7–10 years	1970	1740
11–14 years	2220	1845
15–18 years	2755	2110
19–50 years	2550	1940
51–59 years	2550	1900
60–64 years	2380	1900
65–74 years	2330	1900
over 75 years	2100	1810
pregnancy		+ 200*
lactation		+ 450–480

*During the last three months of pregnancy.

● From Table 3.1, identify the age at which males require the most dietary energy. Suggest why this may be so.

○ The highest energy intake, 2755 kcal per day, is required between the ages of 15 and 18. This is the age range in which boys grow and increase their muscle mass to achieve their adult size and shape. They are also maturing sexually at this stage.

Dietary reference values in fact comprise three numbers: the EAR, just discussed, the reference nutrient intake, RNI, and the lower reference nutrient intake, LRNI. These figures replace the old recommended daily amount (RDA), which was felt not to offer sufficient flexibility for individuals' differing needs. The RNI is set at a level that satisfies the requirements of 97.5% of the population, and the LRNI is set at a level that satisfies the needs of only 2.5% of the population. Thus almost everyone has requirements falling between these two figures. You may have noticed that over the last few years the information on food packaging has shifted emphasis from a categorical 'satisfies 20% of RDA', for example, and more towards a list of ingredients, perhaps with an exhortation to 'eat five portions of fruit each day'. This reflects the move away from a 'one-size-fits-all' RDA to a situation in which individuals' needs can be accommodated.

Individual requirements for nutrients vary considerably depending on factors such as age and sex as you saw above. Other relevant factors are size, metabolic rate (see below) and occupation. The situation is further complicated as interactions between components of the diet may alter the efficiency of absorption or utilization of a particular nutrient. The body also has stores of certain nutrients (fat-soluble vitamins, for example) so that variations in daily intake of such nutrients can be accommodated. Thus it could be misleading to recommend a particular daily intake level.

Summary of Section 3.2.1

1   A balanced diet consists of six main nutrient groups; proteins, carbohydrates, lipids, vitamins, minerals and water.

2   Dietary reference values (DRVs) comprise a range and an estimated average of recommended daily intake levels for nutrients and energy for males and females at different stages of their life.

3.2.2 Balanced energy intake

There is a need for a certain daily energy intake to allow metabolism to occur in the body. **Metabolism** means all the chemical reactions occurring in the body and there are two types of process involved: **catabolism** breaks down larger molecules into smaller ones often with energy release and **anabolism** is the building up of larger molecules from smaller precursors, often requiring energy. The body requires energy to power anabolic, mechanical (for example, muscle contraction and cellular movement), and transport (for example, the movement of substances across cell membranes) work within the body.

As mentioned in Section 2.5.2, there is an 'energy currency' used by the body in the same way that society uses money, known as adenosine triphosphate or ATP. ATP is represented in Figure 3.2 and is synthesized when certain nutrients are catabolized by the body. You do not need to remember the structure of ATP, but do note the three phosphate groups (*tri*phosphate) and the adenosine group of the molecule – these give it the name of adenosine triphosphate.

Energy is released from ATP when it loses a phosphate group and becomes adenosine *di*phosphate or ADP. The energy released from this ATP catabolism can be used to power the energy-requiring processes in the body. So, using the money analogy, ATP is synthesized (or earned like money) and then catabolized (spent)

Figure 3.2   (a) The structure of ATP. The adenosine part of the molecule, on the left, consists of adenine attached to the sugar ribose. This structure is also found in nucleic acids. Attached to the other end of the ribose sugar is a chain of three phosphate groups. The last of these three, at the extreme right of the ATP molecule, is the one that can detach, releasing the energy stored in its chemical bond. The released phosphate group is known as 'P$_i$'. (b) The relationship between ATP, ADP, P$_i$ and energy.

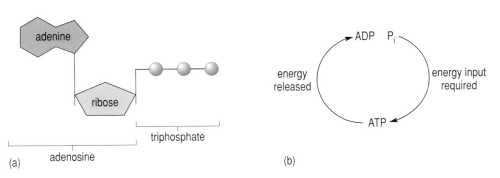

where necessary. There is a difference in the analogy here in that the body is very efficient in how it uses ATP and wastes as little as possible, whereas we are not always as wise in the way we spend money! Proteins, carbohydrates and fats can all be catabolized to produce ATP. The metabolism of these macromolecules involves quite complicated biochemical pathways to ensure that the maximum amount of ATP is synthesized from each starting molecule. Figure 3.3 shows these pathways in a greatly simplified manner, although we do appreciate that they will not look simple if you have not previously studied biology! Note that ATP cannot be stored in the cell, so a constant supply of raw materials is necessary to maintain supplies.

Energy is released when certain nutrients are metabolized in the body and this energy is used to power other chemical reactions and cellular processes while some energy is lost as heat. Energy is measured in kilocalories (kcal) or kilojoules (kJ): one kcal is approximately 4.2 kJ and is defined as the amount of energy required to raise the temperature of 1 litre of water by 1 °C. Electrically igniting known quantities of the foodstuff in oxygen and then measuring the heat output gives an indication of the energy content of foods. The heat energy that is released by burning the food in oxygen is equivalent to the energy released in the body when the complex molecules in the food are metabolized completely. One of the reasons why metabolic pathways are so long and complex is that this allows a gradual release of the energy from the food rather than a sudden

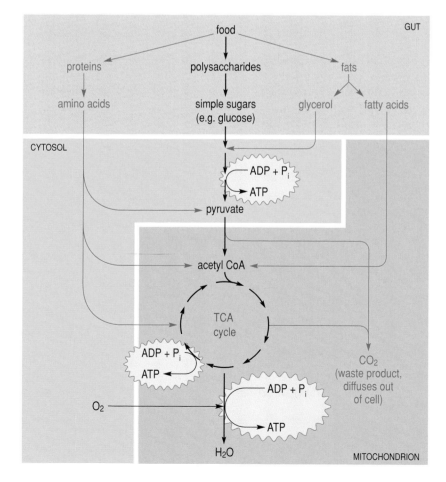

Figure 3.3   Summary of the fates of proteins, carbohydrates and fats in metabolic pathways that result in the production of ATP. Food in the gut is broken down into its constituent amino acids, sugars, fatty acids and glycerol, and these building blocks are absorbed into cells. The first time ATP is made is in the cytosol, from sugars or glycerol. An important intermediate, called pyruvate, is made (amino acids can be converted into pyruvate too). Pyruvate is transported into the mitochondrion, where it is converted into acetyl CoA, which is a very important molecule. Fatty acids and amino acids can also be converted into acetyl CoA, Acetyl CoA enters a pathway called the TCA cycle, where more ATP is made. Waste carbon dioxide (CO_2) is also produced at this stage (as it is from the pyruvate into acetyl CoA conversion earlier). Other products of the TCA cycle are further processed to make more ATP, and this step requires oxygen (O_2) (the O_2 we breathe in) and produces water (H_2O) as a waste product.

massive energy release, as occurs with burning. The energy yields of different nutrients are shown in Table 3.2.

Table 3.2 The energy yields of different nutrients.

Nutrient type	Available energy/	
	kcal g^{-1}	kJ g^{-1}
carbohydrate	4	15–17
fat	9	37
protein	4	16

● How many times more energy in kJ per gram (kJ g^{-1}) does fat yield than protein?

● Fat yields 37 kJ g^{-1} of energy and protein yields 16 kJ g^{-1} of energy. So fat yields 37÷16 or 2.3 times more energy per gram than protein.

In other words, fats contain a more concentrated form of energy. It is therefore easy to exceed the DRVs for energy when eating a high-fat diet, and the excess is stored as fat in the body. Diets containing high proportions of fats have also been linked with disease (e.g. cancer of the colon and cardiovascular disease). If other energy sources in the diet are insufficient, first stored fat and then proteins are catabolized to provide energy and this will ultimately lead to muscle wasting (as muscles are made of protein).

The **basal metabolic rate (BMR)** is the amount of energy required to carry out the basic processes of life – the processes that continue as you sit quietly or lie asleep, such as breathing and the beating of your heart. BMR values are remarkably constant when related to lean body mass although BMR does change with the age and sex of the individual.

● What evidence have you seen for this variation in BMR with age and sex?

● Table 3.1 shows how EAR varies with these two factors.

Further energy expenditure is necessary to carry out everyday activities beyond the energy required for the BMR; this is called the **total energy expenditure (TEE)**. TEE is directly related to the total amount of muscular activity but also to brain activity (the brain normally uses 20% of the available glucose and oxygen), age, environmental temperature (metabolism increases in cold climates to maintain body temperature), disease (metabolic rate increases by about 8% for every 0.5 °C increase in fever), pregnancy and lactation and energy intake (metabolic rate is decreased in prolonged under-nutrition). An individual maintains a stable weight when their *total energy intake* (TEI) balances their TEE.

● Can you think what a diet containing insufficient energy-producing nutrients for an individual's TEE over a period of months may lead to?

● If TEI is less than TEE over a period of months then the individual will lose body mass (weight). The extent of the weight loss depends on the difference between energy intake and expenditure and if this diet were maintained it would lead to malnutrition and an increased susceptibility to ill-health.

● What would over-consumption of energy-producing nutrients result in?

● Over-consumption would lead to weight gain (largely because of an increase in stored body fats) and eventually to obesity.

Obesity is greatly elevated body weight, above the desirable level, to an extent which is associated with serious increased risk to health. Average energy requirements for males and females at different ages were shown in Table 3.1 and Table 3.3 shows energy expended during different activities for a 70 kg person.

Table 3.3 Energy expenditure per hour during different activities for a 70 kg person.

Form of activity	Energy expended/kcal h^{-1}
lying still, awake	77
sitting at rest	100
typing rapidly	140
dressing or undressing	150
walking on level at 4.8 km h^{-1}	200
jogging at 9 km h^{-1}	570

Our diet and our lifestyle are the main influences on our weight; although there is an additional genetic influence (see Book 4). A simple calculation called the **body mass index** (**BMI**) indicates whether an adult is a healthy weight for their height. To calculate your BMI divide your weight (in kg) by your height (in metres) squared.

$$\mathrm{BMI} = \frac{\text{weight/kg}}{(\text{height/m})^2}$$

There is not one perfect weight for every height but a range that allows for people's build. However, the BMI formula is not suitable for pregnant women, children and some medical conditions. Even with these caveats the BMI is not infallible but it can be a useful guide (Table 3.4).

Table 3.4 Body mass indexes and the associated classifications.

Body mass index	Classification
less than 18.5	underweight
18.5–25	desirable or healthy range
25–30	overweight
30–35	obese (Class I)
35–40	obese (Class II)
over 40	morbidly or severely obese (Class III)

● What is the BMI of a woman of 1.7 m who weighs 65 kg?

● $\dfrac{65}{1.7^2} = \dfrac{65}{1.7 \times 1.7} = \dfrac{65}{2.89} = 22.49$

This value means that she would be in the healthy range for her body mass index.

Both overweight and obesity classifications are associated with increased incidence of serious conditions such as high blood pressure (hypertension), cardiovascular disease and type 2 diabetes (Figure 3.4; see Case Report 3.1), as well as conditions that are not life-threatening, but which do affect well-being, such as varicose veins and arthritis. On the gloomy side, both underweight and overweight individuals have an increased risk of premature death, as shown in Figure 3.5.

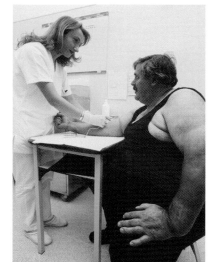

Figure 3.4 A blood sample being taken from the arm of an obese man. The removed blood can then be tested for conditions such as type 2 diabetes.

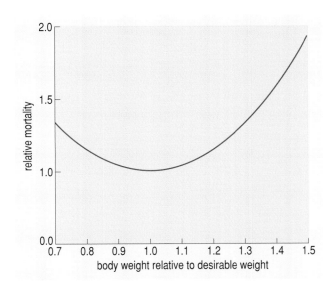

Figure 3.5 The relationship between actual body weight relative to desirable weight and relative mortality.

Inadequate intake

In the developed world inadequate intake of food, at least in terms of energy, is not common. Nevertheless, in many parts of the world starvation is a huge issue, and it is estimated that tens of millions of people face starvation, and well over 5 million, mainly children, die each year from inadequate nutrient intake. Importantly, lack of particular nutrients impairs our ability to carry out many functions.

● Can you suggest any processes that would be impaired by starvation?

● Growth, tissue repair and resistance to infection are all adversely affected by inadequate food intake (Chapter 2).

Thus, people who are starving, or even those who are apparently eating sufficient quantities of food but do not eat a balanced diet, may be susceptible to a variety of illnesses. It is no coincidence that huge increases in the incidence of diseases such as HIV–AIDS and tuberculosis are seen in countries where food is not plentiful, and many starving children are killed by relatively minor ailments that their better-fed counterparts can withstand.

Illness itself can be a cause of inadequate food intake. We all know that illness is often accompanied by a loss of appetite, and if this condition persists, malnutrition can ensue. A lack of appetite is called anorexia, and, ironically, it can also be caused by medical treatment, and by conditions such as depression, particularly in the elderly. In the UK, **anorexia nervosa** is sometimes seen. Anorexia nervosa is a condition manifested by an extreme aversion to food. It might be accompanied by bulimia nervosa, a condition in which the individual binges and then gets rid of the excess food by means of vomiting or laxatives. The disorder usually affects females in the period from their teens until their 30s; only some 5% of anorexic individuals are male.

Psychological hypotheses about the causation of anorexia nervosa fall into three broad categories:

- *Emotional.* Theorists have proposed that some adolescent girls past puberty are trying to regain their childhood body form; anorexic women fail to start to menstruate or cease menstruation with onset of the disorder. Depression and anxiety are common amongst people with anorexia nervosa.

- *Familial.* Families can put too much pressure on children to succeed or may be over protective. Sometimes, the only way an individual can feel 'in charge' of their life is to control their own diet, and this may be manifested by a refusal (overt or tacit) to eat adequate nutrients.

- *Cultural.* Many people have a distorted view of how they should look. People who have anorexia nervosa may compare themselves with what they see as being society's ideal form. Slim young women are used as models in the media and young girls try to emulate them. It is eminently clear that people with anorexia nervosa have a distorted psychological image of their own body. Ironically, it is believed to be the case that many fashion models are suffering from inadequate food intake and that there is a price to be paid for their extremely thin appearance.

Obesity

At the time of writing (2004) 20% of the adult population of the UK is classified as obese. The number of obese children has doubled since 1982, 10% of six year olds and 17% of fifteen year olds are now classified as obese. As shown in Table 3.4, obesity is recognized when the BMI exceeds 30 and occurs quite simply when energy intake exceeds energy expended over a period of time. However, hormonal, genetic and metabolic abnormalities can also sometimes be involved. (We will return to a consideration of these factors in Book 4.) Some obese people eat considerably more than non-obese people, particularly in the period during which they are actually increasing in weight. However, the difference between intake and metabolic expenditure need only be very small (perhaps eating an extra piece of cake every day for 3 months) to produce a cumulative weight increase over a period of months.

The House of Commons Health Committee published a report in 2004 (House of Commons Health Committee, 2004) in which the increasing problem of obesity was heavily emphasized. The report stated that the incidence of obesity has grown by almost 400% in 25 years and suggested that if it continued to grow at such a rate it would soon overtake smoking as the biggest cause of premature loss of life. The economic cost of obesity was estimated at 3.3–3.7 billion pounds per year. This cost estimate includes predicted costs of the NHS for treatment of obese patients as well as time lost to industry due to sickness.

The report makes many recommendations to government of ways of tackling obesity. Targeting the food industry to reduce food portion sizes and moderate their advertising campaigns were some of the recommendations. The report also recommended that food products were labelled more clearly and a 'traffic light' method for labelling foods based on their *energy density* was suggested. In this system 'green' would label foods with low energy, 'amber' for medium energy density and 'red' for high energy density.

- What do you suppose is meant by 'high energy density'?
- A food with high energy density will make available far more energy for its size (i.e. per portion) than a low-energy-density food.

- What happens if the amount of energy that can be made available exceeds current requirements?
- The surplus will be stored, potentially adding to body fat.

Education of what constitutes a healthy diet was also a key recommendation, at school level and beyond. There were a number of different recommendations of ways in which to increase individuals' exercise to the recommended level of 30 minutes five times a week, including school and workplace initiatives.

Exercise is very helpful in aiding obese individuals to lose weight as it increases their TEE. Exercise also has the advantage of increasing BMR for hours beyond the termination of exercise. A long-term advantage of exercise can be an increase in the ratio of lean/fat body weight with subsequent advantages for keeping metabolic rate high. Whilst it is desirable for obese individuals to exercise this is easier said than done and the danger is that individuals can get into a vicious circle: as weight increases so exercise decreases. This means that later, even with the will to do it, an overweight person might not be able to perform enough exercise to increase metabolism sufficiently to lose weight.

There are of course various social, economic and environmental factors that will play a role in how much exercise a person is able to take.

- From your general knowledge summarize some of these factors.
- Your summary should be a long one! It might also reflect your age and current interests. Social factors could include family responsibilities, the availability of others to participate in team games or how close you are to clubs and leisure facilities. Economic factors such as cost of membership of clubs and of sporting equipment and sports wear will limit participation by some people. Even walking, which can be a solitary activity and need not involve the outlay of any cash can be limited if one lives in an unsafe environment.

The relationship between decreased physical activity and increasing obesity within the population of the UK can be attributed to a reduction in cycling and walking and increased car use (the number of cars has doubled in 30 years) and increased television viewing (which has also doubled since the 1960s).

- Is the relationship between decreased physical activity, increased car ownership and obesity a causal relationship?
- The report is suggesting that it is.

- Do you have any reservations about this statement?
- Yes, you should. In the absence of specific data from studies that have eliminated other possible causal factors it is not possible to make inferences about causation just using a common sense approach. (Remember the surprising findings of the Southampton Group cited in Chapter 1.) We will consider this further in Book 4.

The rise in the number of obese children has been associated with increased television watching, playing of computer games and safety fears of parents for their children which keeps them indoors rather than playing outside. The rise of the 'school run' in which children are transported to school rather than walking also does not help with increasing their physical activity levels.

● It is known that many obese children have obese parents. What explanations might be given for this effect?

● Either a genetic factor or an environmental factor, or both, could be involved.

● How would you distinguish between these two explanations?

● It would be possible to follow up genetically identical (monozygotic) twins who were separated after birth and brought up in different families.

These kinds of studies have been undertaken and we will consider them in Book 4.

Case Report 3.1 provides a more in-depth look into some of the causes and treatment of obesity.

Case Report 3.1 Obesity

Ron is 59 years old and looking forward to retiring from his sedentary desk job. He was aware that he had gained weight over a number of years and that his weight had increased more rapidly after he sprained his ankle refereeing rugby (causing his retirement from the game) a couple of years ago. He had meant to join the local gym or take up golf but had not quite got around to doing it. He was looking forward to all the time he would have to get fit again once he had retired, as the most exercise he did every day was walk to and from the bus stop to catch the bus to work, which was about 200 yards from his front door.

Ron noticed that he was starting to get breathless when he had to go upstairs and that he had developed varicose veins. He noticed that he frequently suffered from heartburn after eating and started to complain to his wife Margaret that he often just did not feel well. Margaret, a slim woman in her mid-fifties, urged him to go and have a check-up. He booked himself into the well person clinic, run by the practice nurse.

Jane, the practice nurse, started the check-up by chatting to Ron about his general health. She asked whether there was any family history of heart disease or strokes and discovered that he was not currently taking any medicines. Ron replied that his father had died of a heart attack when he was 67 years old and his mother had died following a stroke at 60 years old.

The nurse asked Ron about his current eating and exercise habits and Ron explained about the sprained ankle and the knock-on effects from that. He admitted that he liked a fried breakfast, enjoyed a canteen-cooked lunch of two courses and a cooked dinner with pudding. The nurse asked if he snacked during the day and Ron said 'No, but I do have a chocolate biscuit with my mid-morning tea and I like to have a pint or two of beer later in the evening often with a bag of crisps'.

Jane weighed Ron (95 kg), measured his height (1.75 m) and then calculated his body mass index (BMI) as:

$$\frac{95}{1.75^2} = 31$$

The BMI reading indicated that Ron was obese (Class I). Jane also measured Ron's waist and hips, explaining that the ratio between waist and hips should not exceed 0.95 for men over 40 years old. She explained that abdominal or central obesity is indicated by a ratio greater than 0.95 in men and 0.85 in women and that this increases the risks of heart disease and **type 2 diabetes**, which is an impairment of insulin activity. She was quick to point out that the possibility that Ron had these diseases would require further investigation before diagnosis could be made. Ron had a central obesity ratio of 0.96.

Jane measured Ron's blood pressure and discovered it was a bit high (blood pressure will be covered in Book 3). Jane pointed out that this reading was a one-off reading and the usual standard for measuring blood pressure is to take one reading per week for 3 weeks. Finally Jane asked Ron to give an urine sample which she tested for glucose (glucosuria is the term used to describe glucose presence in the urine) and ketones (ketones or ketone bodies are a by-product of metabolism when there is excess glucose and ketonuria is the term used to describe the presence of ketones in the urine). Ron's urine sample was negative for glucose and ketones. Glucosuria and ketonuria are indicative of type 2 diabetes.

Jane then asked if Ron had ever considered losing weight and Ron said he would like to but did not know where to start. Jane suggested that Ron kept a diary of his daily food intake and his exercise over the next week and brought it to the next appointment. She told Ron that obesity is caused by taking in more energy than is expended over a period of time and reassured Ron that if he lost weight he would immediately start reducing the risks of the other conditions associated with obesity. She stressed that obesity is a condition that Ron himself could have some control over by eating a balanced diet and increasing his exercise. Ron left the surgery determined to enrol in a local WeightWatchers group and join the gym.

Obesity treatment

Obesity treatment is only successful if weight is reduced and maintained to within a desired range. There are three approaches to obesity treatment: changing behaviour and diet is the most common approach although drugs and surgery can be used in some severe cases of obesity.

Behaviour and diet: it is important to be realistic about an obese patient's target weight as many patients have over-ambitious targets that they are unlikely to achieve. A severely obese patient probably cannot reach an ideal BMI quickly (losing too much weight too quickly puts metabolic stress on the body), but even a weight loss of 10% body weight can significantly reduce the risk of obesity-related disorders. The best combination for weight loss is increasing exercise and decreasing food intake and for lasting effects of obesity treatment a change in eating and exercise habits is necessary and most effective.

Exercise must be based around activities the patient enjoys and can fit into their lifestyle and any increase in exercise is better than no exercise at all. Exercise is beneficial in a weight-loss plan because it uses calories and also increases resting metabolic rate afterwards. Most people also experience a feeling of well-being following exercise and this can be a motivating factor to the patient.

Weight loss is not a simple procedure for most people and requires a dogged determination on behalf of the dieter to stick to the desired regime. People losing weight need support and encouragement to adapt to their recommended dietary and behavioural changes. The motivation for women to lose weight is often their own physical appearance, whereas men are more motivated by health concerns. Partners and friends of the person losing weight can help by providing positive support and motivation and emphasizing the benefits of weight loss such as increased stamina, mobility and self-confidence as well as decreased risk of coronary heart disease, strokes, diabetes, etc.

A practice nurse may suggest that a personalized diet plan is made considering the weight, age and activity level and could include the following:

- include fruit and vegetables with meals;
- avoid high-density-energy between-mealtime snacks and replace crisps and chocolate with fruit;
- spread low fat margarine thinly on wholemeal bread;
- eat low-fat products instead of full-fat products;
- do not fry food; instead bake it in the oven or boil it;
- use skimmed milk instead of full-fat milk;
- remove fat from meat and skin from chicken;
- reduce salt intake (this affects water retention: Book 3, Chapter 1);
- do not add sugar to drinks and avoid soft sugary drinks;
- do not eat pastry, cakes or biscuits as part of a daily routine;
- reduce alcohol intake to national guideline levels (alcohol is high in kcal);
- start walking for an hour or 10 000 steps every day.

Drugs: the only drugs licensed for obesity treatment in the UK are sibutramine (Meridia™) which is an appetite suppressant and orlistat which causes fat malabsorption. Drugs are only licensed for those with a BMI greater than 30 and then only after at least 3 months supervised exercise and behaviour modification has failed to achieve weight loss.

Surgery: surgery can be used to treat Class III obesity, although this is not commonly undertaken in the UK. Either the absorptive capacity of the small intestine is reduced by surgically by-passing part of the small intestine or the size of the stomach is reduced (gastric reduction) so limiting the amount of food that can be taken in. There are considerable risks associated with surgery as it puts a strain on the heart and this risk is increased in obese patients. Some patients have their jaws wired which limits the rate and consistency (i.e. texture) of food intake.

Summary of Section 3.2.2

1   There is a need for a certain level of daily energy intake to allow the body to maintain its BMR, and to carry out work.

2   Adenosine triphosphate (ATP) is the chemical currency of energy used by the body and is produced from the metabolism of food.

3   The body mass index or BMI indicates whether an adult is a healthy weight for their height.

4   Inadequate nutrition is a huge problem globally. Anorexia nervosa is one example of inadequate nutrition seen in the UK.

5   Obesity is an increasing problem in the western world and is associated with a number of other medical disorders, such as cardiovascular disease.

3.3 Carbohydrates

Carbohydrates are a large group of compounds and include sugars, starch and fibre. The Department of Health recommended in 1991 that carbohydrates should be the major source of energy in the human diet, providing 50–60% of the daily kilocalories or kilojoules needed.

●   Carbohydrates are found in a variety of foods. From your general knowledge and reading of food labels can you name any foods that are high in carbohydrates?

●   You may have thought of: table sugar, bread, cereals, cakes, pasta and potatoes.

There are two major types of dietary carbohydrate: the polysaccharides (non-sweet) and the monosaccharides and disaccharides (sweet) or so-called simple sugars (sometimes also called free sugars).

Carbohydrates are chemical compounds consisting of the elements carbon (C), hydrogen (H) and oxygen (O) in a 1 carbon: 2 hydrogen: 1 oxygen ratio, i.e. 1C:2H:1O. The simplest form in which a carbohydrate can exist is as a **monosaccharide** (*mono-* means one). There are three monosaccharides that are important in the human diet: glucose, galactose and fructose. These monosaccharides have the molecular formula $C_6H_{12}O_6$ and they are known as

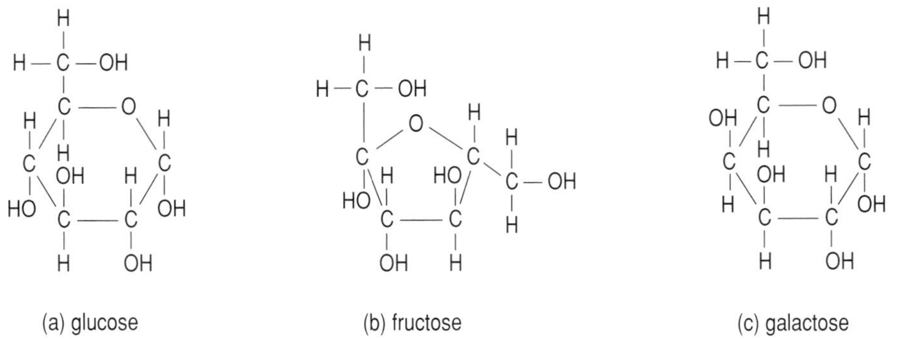

Figure 3.6 Structural formulae for glucose, fructose and galactose.

(a) glucose   (b) fructose   (c) galactose

hexoses (*hex-* means six), which means that they contain 6 carbon atoms, 12 hydrogen atoms and 6 oxygen atoms. The chemical structures of glucose, fructose and galactose are shown in Figure 3.6. You are not expected to remember these structures but do look closely at the formulae to see how the same number of carbon, hydrogen and oxygen atoms are bonded together to give a different overall structure. This is an example of **isomerism**, the existence of two or more chemical compounds containing the same number and type of atoms, but in different arrangements. Glucose, fructose and galactose are known as isomers. Isomerism is common in biological molecules.

● From Figure 3.6, what is the structural difference between glucose and galactose?

○ The H and OH groups attached to the C at the extreme left of the molecule are the opposite way round. The OH is pointing upwards in galactose and downwards in glucose.

When two monosaccharides link together, a **disaccharide** (*di-* means two) is formed and when many monosaccharides link together a **polysaccharide** (*poly-* means many) is formed. For example, sucrose (table sugar) is a disaccharide made up of one glucose and one fructose molecule, and lactose (which is found in milk) is made up of one glucose and one galactose molecule (Figure 3.7).

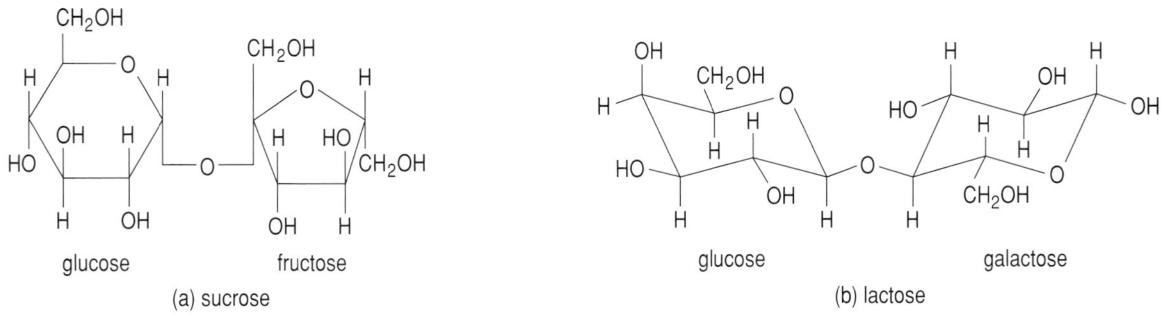

glucose   fructose   glucose   galactose

(a) sucrose   (b) lactose

Figure 3.7 Structural formulae of two disaccharides, (a) sucrose and (b) lactose. The ring carbon atoms and some bonds between atoms have been omitted, which is a commonly used convention. (Note that in (a) the bonds to the O atom linking the constituent hexoses are not really bent!) The representation used in (b) is more informative because it shows the actual shape of the molecule. Note how the molecules are the same as the constituent monosaccharides (glucose and fructose in sucrose and glucose and galactose in lactose) apart from 2 hydrogen atoms and 1 oxygen atom, which are missing in each case. These atoms combine together to give H_2O (water) when the disaccharide is formed.

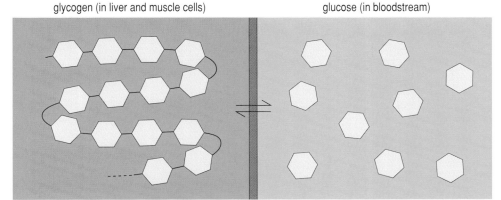

glycogen (in liver and muscle cells)   glucose (in bloodstream)

Figure 3.8   Schematic representation of the interconversion of glucose and glycogen in the body.

Polysaccharides can contain thousands of monosaccharide units. The main polysaccharide found in the human diet is a polymer of glucose called **starch**, which is derived from plants and is found in potatoes, cereals, etc. (**Polymers** are chemical compounds composed of repetitive units.) Animals also have an energy storage polysaccharide called **glycogen**, which is also made up of glucose molecules though in a different arrangement of units. Glycogen is stored in the liver and muscle and can be broken down into its constituent glucose molecules when the body requires energy, as illustrated in Figure 3.8.

● Why would it be useful to store glycogen in muscles?

○ The energy requirements of muscles can increase very rapidly, for example if you suddenly sprint to catch a bus, and the energy molecule ATP cannot be stored. Converting glycogen into glucose *in situ* is the most efficient way of providing fuel for conversion into ATP.

Polysaccharides and disaccharides are too large to be absorbed from the gut and must be broken down into their constituent monosaccharides within the gut.

● Why does eating a chocolate bar result in an almost immediate burst of energy whereas the same energy burst does not arise from eating an equally calorific baked potato?

○ Potatoes contain starch which is a polysaccharide and so needs to be broken down into its constituent glucose molecules before it can be absorbed into the blood, whereas chocolate is packed full of glucose which is more readily absorbed from the gut, causing blood glucose levels to rise more rapidly after ingestion.

3.3.1 Simple sugars

Simple sugars are sweet, soluble monosaccharides or disaccharides. The monosaccharides glucose and particularly fructose are made by plants as sources of energy and stored around their seeds, in the flesh of fruits. Both these monosaccharides are also found in honey. Fructose contains the same amount of energy as glucose (17 kJ or 4 kcal per gram), but tastes twice as sweet and so can be used by those who like sweet foods but are trying to reduce their energy or carbohydrate intake (slimmers or people with diabetes, for example). The most common disaccharide in the diet is sucrose, which is obtained from sugar beet or sugar cane. This sugar is used extensively in manufactured foods. The disaccharide lactose forms about 7% of human milk and about 5% of cows' milk.

Simple sugars can be classified into two groups:

- **intrinsic sugar**, defined as sugar that is contained within the structure of the foodstuff (i.e. in the tough, polysaccharide walls of the plant cells which make up the food material), and usually called dietary fibre.

- **extrinsic sugar**, defined as any sugars not contained within the structure of the foodstuff. Thus extrinsic sugars include those that have been extracted from fruits and those in honey and table sugar as well as the sucrose that is so often added to processed foods.

Lactose (milk sugar) in milk and milk products can be excluded from the latter group as it does not seem to have the same effects on human health as sucrose. For dietary recommendations, the term 'non-milk extrinsic' sugar is therefore used for extrinsic sugars excluding lactose. This classification may seem to be confusing but the two types of sugar (intrinsic and non-milk extrinsic) are thought to have different effects on human health. Intrinsic sugars are thought to have no adverse effects on health, whereas consumption of large amounts of non-milk extrinsic sugars is associated with health risks. For example, such risks include obesity, tooth decay and elevated levels of blood glucose, insulin and cholesterol, which *may* lead to increased incidence of type 2 diabetes and cardiovascular disease. The mechanisms causing these deleterious effects are not fully understood.

The DRVs and actual average intake for carbohydrates are shown in Table 3.5.

Table 3.5   Dietary reference values (DRVs) and actual average intakes of digestible carbohydrates. (Values are per cent of total dietary energy intake; COMA, 1991).

Carbohydrate type	DRV/% total	Average intake/% total
intrinsic sugar, lactose and starch	39	24
non-milk extrinsic sugar	11	18
total	50	42

● From Table 3.5, what can you say about the average person's diet?

◐ Overall, less than 50% of the average dietary intake is coming from carbohydrates. Despite this the average diet contains less intrinsic sugar, lactose and starch than is recommended, and more non-milk extrinsic sugar than is recommended.

● From your own experience, and from your observation of food labels, suggest likely sources of the excess of extrinsic sugars in *your* diet.

◐ Sugars are a major component of many processed foods, but in many cases, food labels do not distinguish between intrinsic and extrinsic sugars. So you may be consuming excess extrinsic sugar without being aware of it. The sources of extra extrinsic sugars have shifted from 'visible' sucrose added by the individual to food and drink, for example you may not add sugar to tea or coffee, to the 'invisible' sources found in processed and manufactured foods.

● Can you suggest why humans (and other animals!) enjoy sugary foods so much?

● Human breast milk is very sweet, so babies may learn to associate satiety and comfort with a sweet taste, an example of a learning process that psychologists call *conditioning*. A 'taste' for sweet foods may have evolved as an adaptive characteristic because fruits were a good source of energy, fibre, vitamins and minerals for the hunter–gatherers (and plants evolved sweet fruits that improved their likelihood of being eaten and their seeds dispersed). Sociological and cultural factors encourage those in the developed world, particularly children, to eat sweet foods.

It is crucial that blood glucose levels of approximately 4–6 millimoles per litre (mmol l^{-1}) are maintained to ensure the delivery of glucose to red blood cells and neurons (nerve cells), as glucose is the only fuel that these cell types can use, except in times of extreme starvation. Glucose is used in the cell as an energy source because its catabolism is linked to the production of ATP, as you saw earlier in Figure 3.3. Thirty-six molecules of ATP are synthesized from the oxidation (catabolism) of each molecule of glucose.

A mole is the unit for an amount of a substance. Here 1 millimole of glucose = 180 mg glucose.

Any absorbed monosaccharides that are not immediately used by cells to produce energy are converted into the polysaccharide storage molecule glycogen, which is stored in liver and muscle cells. Glycogen can be converted back into glucose and then released into the blood to provide energy at times when glucose is not being absorbed from the gut. When there is a large excess these carbohydrates are converted into triacylglycerols (fats).

● Where are fats stored?

● Fats are stored in the special fat storage cells in adipose tissue.

Triacylglycerols can be broken down to release fatty acids into the blood, and many cells can use these as an energy source instead of glucose.

It is possible that the elevated levels of blood glucose that occur in individuals who regularly *overeat* very sugary foods, may lead to over-stimulation and, in the long-term, a disruption of the normal control system that regulates blood glucose (Book 2, Chapter 3). This may be one of the reasons why overweight individuals are more prone than those of 'desirable' weight to develop type 2 diabetes.

3.3.2 Polysaccharides

The main polysaccharides that we consume are starch, glycogen and cellulose and all three of these are composed only of glucose molecules, though in different arrangements. Glycogen, found in meat, is the carbohydrate storage compound of animals and is digestible by humans. Starch and cellulose are plant polysaccharides: starch is the storage compound of plants and is mostly digestible by humans, whereas cellulose is a structural component of plant cell walls and cannot be digested by humans. Cellulose is a non-starch polysaccharide (NSP; see Table 3.6) that plays an important role in our diet as it contributes to the non-digestible part of our food called fibre or roughage. Cellulose is insoluble in water and hence known as insoluble fibre. The two other types of fibre are *pectins* from fruit and *mucilages* from pulses (peas and beans). These form a jelly-like structure in water and are known as soluble fibre.

Table 3.6   Non-starch polysaccharide (NSP) content of some common foods. Adapted from Englyst et al. (1988).

Food	Total NSP (g per 100 g)
white bread	1.5
wholemeal bread	5.8
weetabix	9.7
white rice	0.2
apples	1.6
banana	1.1
peanuts	6.2
baked beans	3.5
potatoes	1.2
carrots	2.5

Starch can be classified into rapidly digestible starch, slowly digestible starch and resistant starch, which is not digested by the human in the small intestine, but by bacteria in the large intestine, resulting in increased faecal volume and flatulence. The relative amounts of different types of starch in a meal can have a significant effect on blood glucose levels after eating that meal; this is one reason why porridge oats or muesli may be a better breakfast cereal than the highly processed and sugared cereals which are so appealing to children. The relatively unprocessed wholegrain cereal (oats) will take longer to be digested than the processed alternative, and will therefore produce a less rapid and smaller rise in blood glucose levels. However, it will continue to be digested and monosaccharides will be absorbed over a longer period of time. A similar effect occurs for pasta (white pasta contains 43% slowly digestible starch), compared with white bread (4% slowly digestible starch).

3.3.3 Carbohydrate-associated disorders

Both insoluble and soluble fibre are thought to be important to a healthy diet. Diets that contain plentiful insoluble fibre result in bulkier gut contents, which, because gut muscle activity is stimulated by the larger volume, travel more quickly through the digestive system, in other words, the food has a reduced *transit time*.

● Can you think of a common disorder that might be treated by increased fibre in the diet?

● Constipation. The transit time for food that is low in fibre can be several days or longer, whereas a meal that is high in insoluble fibre can pass through the gut in about a day.

In fact NSP foods can be used as *bulk purgatives* to loosen the bowel in cases of constipation.

A shortened transit time reduces the amount of contact between intestinal tissue and any potentially harmful substances in the diet. Fibre may also actually bind potentially toxic substances, and hence aid their elimination via defaecation. For this reason, it is thought that diets high in insoluble fibre are protective against conditions such as bowel cancer, and indeed, the incidence of bowel cancer is lower in populations with a higher intake of insoluble fibre. Diets high in fibre are also associated with a lower incidence of diabetes and heart disease and as they also tend to be low in fat and sugar, and in some cases have higher levels of some vitamins, there may be further beneficial effects.

Bulky food also reduces the need for straining at defaecation, which can cause piles or haemorrhoids (dilated veins causing painful swelling at the anus). Diets containing high levels of insoluble fibre have also been reported to have a protective effect against some other gastrointestinal disorders, including formation of gallstones (the small stone-like structures formed when cholesterol solidifies in the gall bladder), appendicitis (inflammation of the appendix), and diverticular disease. Diverticular disease is a gastrointestinal disorder in which areas of the gut wall are deformed into small 'pockets' called diverticula. The formation of diverticula is thought to occur when the walls of the intestine are pushing against gut contents, which are hard and compacted, as occurs with low-fibre diets. Gut contents become stuck in these pockets, so allowing infection. Eventually these sections of the gut become painful and inflamed.

The proportion of the different types of starch in the diet is very important for people with diabetes, who cannot regulate blood glucose levels. You read in Section 3.3.1 that elevated levels of glucose in the circulation can be harmful; a major reason for this is that when glucose is present at high levels, it can bind to proteins (this is known as glycation). This binding causes irreversible structural changes to the protein and the formation of what is known as **Amadori product.** This compound can bind irreversibly to other proteins, resulting in long-term damage to blood vessels such as those in the retina of the eye which can lead to blindness, peripheral nerve damage and connective tissue damage in the elderly. It is important to note that although protein glycation is a major problem for untreated diabetics, it also occurs in individuals without diabetes, though at a lower level.

Summary of Section 3.3

1   The Department of Health recommends that carbohydrates are the major source of energy in our diet.

2   Carbohydrates are a large chemical group consisting of monosaccharides (e.g. glucose and fructose), disaccharides (e.g. lactose and sucrose) and polysaccharides (e.g. starch and glycogen).

3   Glucose is maintained at a concentration of approximately 4–6 mmol l^{-1} in the blood, as it is an essential energy molecule for the brain and nervous system.

4   Excess glucose is stored as the polysaccharide glycogen in the liver and muscles, and as triacylglycerols in adipose cells.

5   Polysaccharides from plant material that cannot be broken down and digested in the gut are called fibre.

6   Fibre exists in soluble and non-soluble forms. High fibre diets are linked to a reduced incidence of colon cancer and other disorders.

7   Excess levels of glucose in the blood lead to the formation of Amadori product. In the long-term this is thought to result in damage to a number of tissues of the body.

3.4 Lipids

Fatty foods taste very pleasant to humans, but fat is often seen as the 'baddie' in modern diet. The Department of Health recommends eating small amounts of fatty foods (Figure 3.1). Fats are defined as being insoluble in water and encompass fats (solid) and oils (liquid). **Lipid** is the chemical name for this food group. The terms 'fats' and 'lipids' tend to be used interchangeably. Table 3.6 (overleaf) shows the total lipid content of a range of foods.

Table 3.6 The lipid content of a range of foods (listed in descending order).

Food	Lipid content/%	Food	Lipid content/%
lard	99	beef (rump steak)	14
butter	82	chicken roast	5.4
margarine	81	salmon, smoked	4.5
cream cheese	47	whole milk	3.9
cheddar cheese	34	rice	1
pork sausage	32	skimmed milk	0.1
smoked mackerel	30.9	potatoes	0.1

Lipids have a range of functions in the body and these are outlined below. Lipids:

- are a concentrated source of energy with 1 gram of fat releasing 37 kJ of energy;

- are stored as triacylglycerols in adipose tissue for times of energy need, such as during exercise, and for other purposes;

- prolong emptying time of the stomach, thereby postponing hunger pangs;

- transport and store fat-soluble vitamins;

- provide a source of **precursors** (building blocks) for cellular structures and signalling molecules;

- insulate neurons by providing the protective fatty sheath around them called myelin;

- include cholesterol (an important membrane component) and some hormones.

It has also been suggested that lipids have a role in protecting and supporting body organs, and also in thermal insulation, but there is little evidence to support these theories, and quite a lot to disprove them (Pond, 1998).

Lipids are not polymers like carbohydrates and proteins, but aggregates of individual lipid molecules which associate together. Lipids are composed of carbon, hydrogen and oxygen atoms, as are carbohydrates, but have a smaller proportion of oxygen than carbohydrates. The fact that lipids contain less oxygen means that the molecules are less able to form polar (or charged) molecules and so do not interact readily with polar water molecules. This property of lipids is known as hydrophobicity (water hating) and explains why water dropped onto a greasy frying pan goes into droplets because the water and oil do not mix.

The major dietary lipids are the triacylglycerols contained in fats and oils, which are made up of three **fatty acid** molecules combined with one molecule of glycerol as illustrated in Figure 3.9.

In Figure 3.9 you can see that one of the fatty acid chains is bent and if you look closely at the bend you will see that it has two chemical bonds between the two carbon (C) atoms. This is known as a 'double bond' and it is very rigid in comparison to a 'single bond' between carbon atoms. Fatty acids without double bonds are known as **saturated fatty acids** and fatty acids with double bonds are known as **unsaturated fatty acids**. Fatty acids with one double bond are known

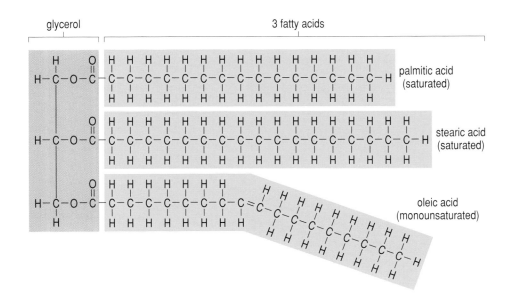

palmitic acid (saturated)

stearic acid (saturated)

oleic acid (monounsaturated)

Figure 3.9   A triacylglycerol molecule. Note the three fatty acid chains and one glycerol molecule. You can see that the saturated fatty acids are so called because they are saturated with hydrogen (H) atoms. There is no possibility of adding further H atoms into this structure.

as **monounsaturated fatty acids** and those with many double bonds are known as **polyunsaturated fatty acids**. Because the chains of unsaturated fatty acids are bent they take up more space and so unsaturated fatty acids are less dense than saturated fatty acids. Fats which are fairly solid contain a higher proportion of saturated fatty acids, whereas less solid fats and liquid oils contain more unsaturated fatty acids. We cannot make fatty acids with double bonds, so must obtain them from the diet.

If you read the nutrition information on a margarine carton it gives you the total fat content per 100 g of the margarine and then breaks down the fat content into the following groups: saturates, monounsaturates, polyunsaturates, omega-3 (or *n*-3) fatty acids, omega-6 (or *n*-6) fatty acids and trans fatty acids. The healthier margarines are the ones with a higher proportion of unsaturated fatty acids.

● Why should people trying to lose weight eat margarine with a higher percentage of polyunsaturated fatty acids?

● Margarine with a higher percentage of polyunsaturated fatty acids is less dense than margarine with saturated fatty acids. This means that for the same *volume*, the margarine containing polyunsaturated fatty acids will contain fewer calories than margarine with saturated fatty acids.

Unsaturated fatty acids are grouped into three series known as omega-3, omega-6 and omega-9, with the number referring to the location of the first double bond within the fatty acid. (Incidentally omega tends to be used in the US whilst you will more often find *n*- used in UK publications.) This pattern of unsaturation in fatty acids is also thought to be important for health. Inuit people have a remarkably low incidence of heart disease even though their traditional diet is very high in fat. Their diet is rich in polyunsaturated omega-3 fatty acids from herring and mackerel and this observation has led to the recommendation that we should eat more oily fish in our diets.

● Some fatty acids are essential nutrients. Can you remember what an essential nutrient is?

● Essential nutrients are molecules that cannot be made by the body and need to be supplied in the diet.

Linoleic (an omega-6 fatty acid) and α-linolenic (an omega-3 fatty acid) acids are essential nutrients and both these fatty acids are needed as components of cellular membranes. They are also required for the synthesis of important signalling molecules called *eicosanoids*, which include the *prostaglandins*. These signalling molecules are made by breaking down certain of the phospholipids in the cell membrane. Other molecules derived from lipids, such as some vitamins, also act as signalling molecules. Linoleic and α-linolenic acids are found in green plants, and particularly in linseed oil from flax.

● Fatty acids are crucial components of cellular membranes as phospholipids (Section 2.5.1). What other kind of fat is important in membranes?

● Cholesterol.

Cholesterol is a lipid which has received a particularly 'bad press', because elevated levels of some forms of cholesterol in plasma have been found to be a risk factor for cardiovascular disease. This is discussed below. However, cholesterol has vital roles in the human body: it is a component of cell membranes and is also a precursor molecule for the manufacture of other molecules such as vitamin D, steroid hormones (Book 2, Chapter 3) and bile salts.

Cholesterol is synthesized by the liver and only 20–25% comes from dietary sources (cholesterol is found at high levels in eggs and animal products such as kidney and liver). Under normal circumstances, if dietary intake is high, there is a corresponding reduction of cholesterol synthesis by the liver. Thus, for most individuals, the amount of cholesterol consumed is unlikely to result in an elevated level of cholesterol found in blood plasma. Cholesterol and fatty acids, being fatty substances, do not readily mix with blood, which is predominantly watery. To get around this problem, they are transported by protein carriers in the blood. The protein-lipid complexes are known as lipoproteins, and their density differs depending on the relative proportions of protein (heavy) and fat (light). There are several classes of lipoproteins, but here we concentrate on the **low-density lipoproteins (LDL)** and **high-density lipoproteins (HDL)**. LDL are composed of 25% protein and 75% lipid and supply cholesterol to cells, and HDL (50% protein and 50% lipid) transport surplus cholesterol from cells to the liver to be broken down or repackaged. The ratio of HDL to LDL is associated with risk of atherosclerosis, the deposition of lipid in arteries (Section 3.4.1): the greater the proportion of HDL the lower the risk. The ratio of HDL to LDL is therefore an important indicator of risk of cardiovascular disease. Fatty acid intake influences blood cholesterol levels, which should be below 5.2 mmol per litre. Unsaturated fatty acids increase the proportion of HDL and thereby lower blood cholesterol levels, whereas saturated fatty acids increase the proportion of LDL and raise blood cholesterol levels.

All this means that the *total* fat intake, and also the *types* of fat in the diet have an effect on plasma cholesterol levels. For this reason, the recommendations for fat intake specify not only the total amount of fat in the diet, but also the relative amounts of the different types of fatty acid, as shown in Table 3.7.

Table 3.7 Dietary reference values (DRVs) for fats and fatty acids and actual intakes as a percentage of total daily energy intake (adult population average in the UK). (The difference in the values for total fats and total fatty acids is accounted for by the energy derived from glycerol.) (COMA, 1991)

	DRV/% total (no alcohol)	DRV/% total (assumes 5% alcohol)	Average actual intake (and range) /% total
total fats	35	33	39 (30–50)
total fatty acids	32.5	30	35
saturated fatty acids	11	10	17 (10–23)
cis-polyunsaturated fatty acids	6.5	6	6*(3–12)
cis-monounsaturated fatty acids	13	12	12*(8–17)
trans-fatty acids	2	2	

* Includes actual intake of *trans*-fatty acids (approximately 2% of total).

● From Table 3.7, what can you say about the actual average intake compared to the recommendations?

◐ On average, we eat much more saturated fatty acids than we should, although our actual intake of polyunsaturated fatty acids complies much more closely with the guidelines.

On inspection of Table 3.7, you will notice two points that we have not yet discussed. First, alcohol is taken into account in the current guidelines for energy intake. (Similar reductions in the recommended contribution of carbohydrates to the total energy intake are made if alcohol is consumed.) This is because alcohol yields a considerable amount of energy: 29 kJ (or 6.9 kcal) per gram.

● How does this yield compare with that of carbohydrate and fat?

◐ Alcohol yields more energy per gram than carbohydrate but less than a gram of fat (see Table 3.2).

The second point to note from Table 3.7 is that recommendations about the amounts of different *types* of unsaturated fatty acids are made. Unsaturated fatty acids can be classified in several ways. One important division is between the fatty acid *isomers*: *cis*- and *trans*- fatty acids. The *cis*-fatty acids have both parts of the hydrocarbon chain on the *same* side of the double bond of the molecule whilst *trans*-fatty acids have parts of the hydrocarbon chain on opposite sides. Figure 3.10 shows the *cis*- and *trans*- forms of the monounsaturated fatty acid, oleic acid.

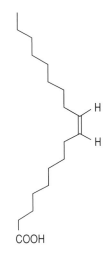

(a) COOH

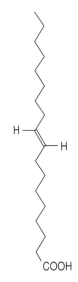

(b) COOH

Figure 3.10 Skeleton formulae of oleic acid isomers: (a) *cis*-oleic acid; (b) *trans*-oleic acid. Skeleton formulae show the shape of organic molecules and only identify atoms or chemical groups of interest; so here the carboxyl (–COOH) groups and the H atoms at the double bonds are shown.

● Predict the relative densities of fats with high *cis-* or high *trans-* isomer content.

● Fats with a high *cis-* content will be less dense (less tightly packed) than fats with a high *trans-* content.

Although this may seem a small structural detail, it is also relevant to the effects that the two types of fatty acid might have on human health. Most naturally occurring fatty acids are in the *cis-* form. Some *trans*-fatty acids are found in fats from ruminant animals (such as sheep and cows) and *trans*-fatty acids are also generated by the food industry in the commonly used process of *hydrogenation*. This is the addition of hydrogen atoms to polyunsaturated fatty acids to make them more saturated and therefore more solid. In this way, an oil is turned into a fat. Hydrogenation increases an oil's stability and also makes it possible to use hardened vegetable oils instead of animal fats for baking, etc. Deep-frying foods in oil also generates *trans*-fatty acids. COMA recommended that *cis*-polyunsaturated fatty acids should make up 6% of total dietary energy, while *trans*-unsaturated acids should make up no more that 2% of dietary energy (Table 3.7).

3.4.1 Lipid-associated disorders

As most lipids can be made from carbohydrates there is a very limited requirement for this food group in our diets.

● What specific requirements are there in relation to fat/lipid intake?

● We have an absolute requirement with respect to the two essential fatty acids. They cannot be made.

● Name the two essential fatty acids.

● Linoleic acid and α-linolenic acid are the two essential fatty acids.

The amounts required are relatively small. The suggested DRVs (COMA, 1991) are that they provide 1% and 0.2% of TEI, respectively. In the developed world this is easily achieved, representing a serving of green vegetables or seed oil used in cooking.

● Why might this surprise some people?

● It might seem unlikely that a portion of green vegetable could provide the total lipid requirement of a diet!

In general fatty foods taste pleasant and so an excess of this food group in a diet is common and, as you saw in Section 3.2.2, excess of any energy-providing nutrient can lead to obesity. Obesity itself predisposes to a number of other conditions, including cardiovascular disease. Cardiovascular disease is a major cause of death in the developed world and contributes to 39% of deaths in England and Wales (Office for National Statistics, 2003). This disease is discussed in more detail in Book 3, but is touched on here in relation to lipid disorders. There is no single cause of cardiovascular disease and some of the associated risk factors are unavoidable: ageing, being male and family history. However, some risk factors can be controlled by the individual and these include: cigarette smoking, high blood pressure, inactivity, type 2 diabetes and being overweight.

Increased levels of cholesterol, triacylglycerol and LDL (all of which are associated with a high overall fat intake) in the blood predispose an individual to cardiovascular disease. High levels of these substances in the blood can lead to **atherosclerosis**, the deposition of lipid in large and medium arteries, resulting in narrowing and occlusion of the blood vessels, as illustrated in Figure 3.11.

Narrowing of an artery means that tissues after the narrowed point do not receive enough blood for any increased requirements of oxygen and glucose, and this can cause an acute **ischaemic** (oxygen-lacking) pain. Narrowing of an artery supplying blood to the heart (a coronary artery) is likely to cause **angina** (pain on exercise) as the heart needs to work harder to pump blood around the body but does not receive the oxygen and glucose it needs. When an artery is totally blocked or occluded the tissues it supplies rapidly die from ischaemia. If a coronary artery is occluded a heart attack occurs whereas occlusion of an artery leading to the brain causes a stroke.

Making small dietary changes is the simplest and most effective way of reducing the risk of cardiovascular disease. Such changes include the following:

- reducing fat intake to no more than 35% of total calorie intake (and of this, fewer than 10% of calories from saturated fats);

- increasing intake of fruit and vegetables that contain vitamins C and E, which have a role as antioxidants (see Section 3.7);

- reducing cholesterol levels by including more wholegrain foods and fibre (fibre increases cholesterol elimination from the gut, and also has a satiating effect, reducing overall eating);

- drinking moderate amounts (up to 2 units a day) of alcohol: moderate amounts of alcohol increase levels of HDL, and some alcoholic drinks such as red wine also contain antioxidants; however, a higher intake of alcohol is associated with a higher risk of cardiovascular disease; interestingly, so is a lower intake!

Summary of Section 3.4

1   Fats are a concentrated form of energy, and give food a pleasant and satisfying taste.

2   Linoleic and α-linolenic acid are essential fatty acids.

3   The lipid cholesterol is an essential component of cell membranes and is also the precursor of steroid hormones.

4   Dietary fatty acids can influence the levels of circulating cholesterol; saturated fatty acids raise, and unsaturated fatty acids lower, levels of cholesterol in the blood.

5   Cardiovascular disease is a major killer in the developed world. Eating a diet without an excess of fat is important in helping reduce the risk of this disease.

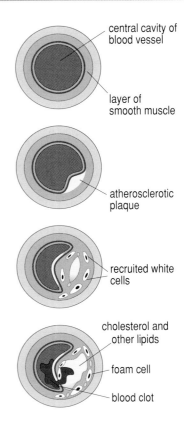

central cavity of blood vessel

layer of smooth muscle

atherosclerotic plaque

recruited white cells

cholesterol and other lipids

foam cell

blood clot

Figure 3.11 Stages in the development of a narrowing blood vessel. Lipids leak from LDL and start to accumulate at particular sites in the blood vessel, called atherosclerotic plaques. A group of white cells is recruited to repair the damage by 'mopping up' the lipid. As they ingest lipid they become bloated with fat and are called foam cells. Eventually they die, and their remains add to the size of the plaque. Meanwhile, the growing plaque interferes more and more with blood flow until the whole vessel may become blocked.

3.5 Proteins

Proteins are an essential component of the human diet and form 12–18% of the total body weight. Their main use is in the growth, repair and maintenance of body tissues. More specifically, for example, enzymes help chemical reactions take place, **antibodies** help combat infection, membrane proteins transport substances across the cell membrane and haemoglobin in red blood cells transports oxygen around the body; these are examples of **globular proteins**. **Fibrous proteins**, such as collagen in bone and the muscle proteins actin and myosin, are involved in structure and support.

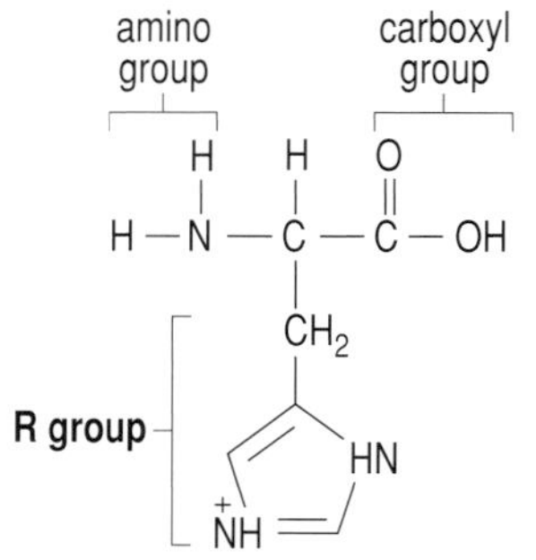

Chemically proteins are polymers made from the elements carbon, hydrogen, oxygen and nitrogen. The building blocks are called amino acids, and there are 20 different amino acids, of which eight are essential; these are another example of an essential nutrient. All the amino acids have a standard type of molecular structure; they contain a carboxyl (COOH) group, an amino (NH₂) group and a side chain or R group, which differs for each amino acid (Figure 3.12). The structure of the R group is crucial because it determines the shape and chemical properties of the amino acid. Table 3.8 shows the 20 amino acids found in proteins. You do not need to learn the amino acid structures but do notice the differences between the amino acids because this is what gives each amino acid its own specific nature.

Figure 3.12 Structure of the amino acid histidine.

● What differences do you notice between the R groups of the amino acids?

○ The R groups differ in shape, size and charge.

Histidine, tyrosine and cysteine are not essential amino acids, but they can only be synthesized from particular essential amino acids. The rest of the non-essential amino acids can be made from a variety of essential amino acids, and by interconversion among themselves. Arginine is made only in small amounts and so must also be included in the diet for young children.

A protein is a polymer of amino acids. The amino acids join together in a chemical reaction, as illustrated in Figure 3.13 where glycine and alanine are linked together to form a dipeptide. The name of the chemical bond between the amino acids is a **peptide bond.**

● From Figure 3.13 decide whether the peptide bond is an example of ionic or covalent bonding.

○ A peptide bond is a covalent bond (Chapter 2).

● The reaction to join two amino acids together is known as a condensation reaction. If you look at Figure 3.13 can you suggest why this is so?

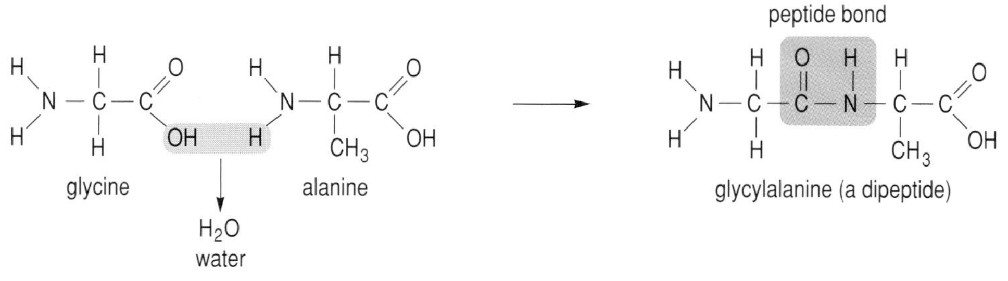

Figure 3.13 How two amino acids join together to form a dipeptide. Note the elimination of a molecule of water in this reaction.

Table 3.8   Amino acids that occur naturally in proteins, grouped according to type of R group. Essential amino acids are indicated with an asterisk.

Amino acid	Symbol	R group	Amino acid	Symbol	R group
aspartate	Asp	COO^- $\mid$ CH_2 $\mid$	alanine	Ala	CH_3 $\mid$
glutamate	Glu	COO^- $\mid$ $(CH_2)_2$ $\mid$	cysteine	Cys	SH $\mid$ CH_2 $\mid$
arginine	Arg	H_2N $\diagdown$ C $\diagup$ $^+NH_2$; NH $\mid$ $(CH_2)_3$ $\mid$	glycine	Gly	H $\mid$
			isoleucine*	Ile	H_3C $\diagdown$ CH $\diagup$ CH_2CH_3 $\mid$
histidine	His	^+NH; HN; CH_2 $\mid$	leucine*	Leu	H_3C $\diagdown$ CH $\diagup$ CH_3; CH_2 $\mid$
lysine*	Lys	$^+NH_3$ $\mid$ $(CH_2)_4$ $\mid$	methionine*	Met	CH_3 $\mid$ S $\mid$ $(CH_2)_2$ $\mid$
asparagine	Asn	$CONH_2$ $\mid$ CH_2 $\mid$	phenylalanine*	Phe	CH_2 $\mid$
glutamine	Gln	$CONH_2$ $\mid$ $(CH_2)_2$ $\mid$	proline	Pro	N—$COOH$; H
serine	Ser	OH $\mid$ CH_2 $\mid$	tryptophan*	Trp	HN; CH_2 $\mid$
threonine*	Thr	OH $\mid$ CH—CH_3 $\mid$			
tyrosine	Tyr	OH; CH_2 $\mid$	valine*	Val	H_3C $\diagdown$ CH $\diagup$ CH_3 $\mid$

negatively charged R groups: aspartate, glutamate

positively charged R groups: arginine, histidine, lysine

uncharged polar R groups: asparagine, glutamine, serine, threonine, tyrosine

non-polar R groups

○ The formation of the peptide bond between the amino acids involves the elimination of a molecule of water, H_2O. This is so called because it is analogous to the 'condensation' that occurs on windows as water vapour in the air changes into liquid water droplets.

Note that the groups involved in this reaction are the carboxyl group and the amino group and that there is a free amino group and carboxyl group on the dipeptide formed. The free carboxyl group can combine with an amino group of another amino acid and so on until a chain of amino acids is formed, creating a protein. So a protein always has an amino end and a carboxyl end, and this is important for function. Proteins synthesized within the cell are made with the amino end first and subsequent amino acids are added to the carboxyl end of the growing chain of amino acids. The number of possible combinations of the 20 amino acids is enormous and it is the different nature of the amino acids and their arrangement within the protein that gives each protein its overall structure and functional characteristics.

Proteins in the diet are derived from the cells of the plants and animals that we eat, and are broken down by the digestive system. The absorbed amino acids are used to make new proteins.

● Proteins are broken down into amino acids. What common chemical is required for this?

○ Water, to break the peptide bonds. (Remember that the formation of these bonds involved the elimination of water.)

There is a constant process of protein synthesis and degradation going on throughout the body.

● Why do we need a constant supply of protein? Couldn't the body simply keep recycling the amino acids in its own proteins?

○ Protein is constantly lost from the body, e.g. via the shedding of skin cells and through bodily secretions (such as digestive juices). Loss is also heavy at times of illness and injury (e.g. loss of blood and damaged tissues as described in Chapter 2).

Table 3.9 shows the protein content of some common foods.

Some foods, such as eggs, milk and beef, contain all the amino acids necessary for the human diet. However, other sources of protein may contain levels of particular amino acids that are insufficient for human requirements, and this can lead to deficiency diseases. This is a particular problem is some less developed regions. For example many communities rely on maize as their principal staple food and maize is deficient in available tryptophan. Some vegetarian and vegan diets are deficient in essential amino acids. Wheat, for example, is low in the amino acid lysine, so anyone choosing to eat a restricted diet should ensure that they do consume sufficient essential amino acids. For people whose diets contain a variety of protein sources, these individual deficiencies in particular foods are not important. For those whose diets are restricted in the variety of protein sources that are used, these deficiencies can cause illness.

Table 3.9 The protein content of some common foods.

Animal-derived foods	Protein content/%	Plant-derived foods	Protein content/%
cheese (cheddar)	26	soya flour (low fat)	45
bacon (lean)	20	soya flour (full fat)	37
beef (lean)	20	peanuts	24
cod	17	bread (wholemeal)	9
herring	17	bread (white)	8
eggs	12	rice	7
beef (fat)	8	peas (fresh)	6
milk	3	potatoes (old)	2
cheese (cream)	3	bananas	1
butter	less than 1	apples	less than 1

Protein intakes in the UK are more than adequate for our needs. Table 3.10 shows the recommended daily intakes of protein for individuals of different ages.

Table 3.10 Dietary reference values (as RNIs) for protein intakes in men and women (COMA, 1991).

Gender and status	RNI/g per day
Males	50
Females	44.5
during pregnancy	+ 6
during lactation:	
baby 0–4 months	+ 11
baby more than 4 months	+ 8

The '+' signs indicate that these values are to be added to the adult requirement.

● Can you think of any people that might need extra dietary protein?

● Extra dietary protein is needed by people who have an injury, infection, burns or cancer, as all of these can result in an increased loss of protein.

● At what stages of life might there also be a requirement for extra dietary protein?

● Women who are pregnant or breastfeeding need a plentiful supply of protein, as do professional athletes in active training.

● Women lose protein via menstruation, yet the requirement for non-pregnant, non-lactating women is lower than that for males. Suggest why this might be so.

● Men generally are larger than women, and have a higher proportion of muscle (which is largely protein) than do women. Thus their requirement for dietary protein is, on average, greater.

3.5.1 Protein-associated disorders

In the developed world most individuals consume in excess of the DRVs. For example, in the UK the National Food Survey 2000 (DEFRA, 2000) gave a value of around 67 g per person per day. By 2003 it was estimated that over 71g per person per day was being consumed. However, these values are way below the suggested upper safe limit of 1.5 g per kg of body weight per day (DoH, 1991). There has subsequently been discussion of whether there are *any* deleterious effects on health from consuming high levels of protein, as it has not been possible to provide clear evidence of negative effects (Manninen, 2004).

On the other hand in the developing world, human diets are often deficient in protein as well as in overall energy content. Protein–energy malnutrition (PEM) is a condition where the diet of adults and children is lacking in a range of nutrients and overall food intake is too low for their bodily requirements.

Marasmus is a severe form of PEM and is a condition that results from a long-term insufficiency in energy intake. It is a condition often seen in famines, although low-level marasmus can occur throughout a vulnerable population, with only the most severe cases being noticed. Once the body's fat stores are depleted, muscle and organ protein is broken down to provide energy. The epithelial cells and villi of the gut are also affected by marasmus and this can lead to poor absorption of nutrients from the inadequate diet. This cycle of inadequate diet and poor absorption of nutrients leads to the severe body wasting that is seen in the victims of famine.

Kwashiorkor is protein deficiency in children. It can occur when children are weaned from breast milk onto protein-poor foods such as cassava (a root vegetable) or green bananas. Repeated childhood infections and a lack of vitamins and minerals exacerbate the condition, which is characterized by **oedema** (swelling due to fluid retention) and a general lack of energy for any activity. Growth stops and there is severe liver damage, loss of weight and pigmentation from skin.

Pellagra (niacin deficiency) is common in parts of Africa and South America where the staple food is maize. Maize (corn) is low in the essential amino acids lysine and tryptophan. Tryptophan is used by the body to make niacin (see Section 3.7.2). Pellagra causes skin lesions, diarrhoea and eventually death if left untreated. In the developed world, maize is eaten (mainly in the form of cornflakes) as part of a *varied* diet; niacin deficiency is therefore very rare in the developed world.

Phenylketonuria (*PKU*) is an inherited condition with an incidence of 1 in 10 000 births in the UK (see Case Report 1.1). The condition prevents the conversion of the amino acid phenylalanine (found in milk) into tyrosine. The accumulation of the phenylalanine causes progressive brain damage. All newborn babies are screened for PKU between 6 and 10 days old by the 'blood spot' test. If a baby is diagnosed with PKU it is treated by diet.

● How would a dietician treat a child with PKU?

◉ The intake of phenylalanine is reduced, but it is still included in the diet to keep levels of this essential amino acid at normal levels. The diet is supplemented by tyrosine.

The dietician would also provide information and support for the family to ensure that the child had sufficient intake of all the other nutrients to allow optimal growth.

Summary of Section 3.5

1   Protein is an essential component of the diet. The eight essential dietary amino acids (together with amino acids synthesized in the body) are used to produce new proteins which replace those continually lost via the shedding of skin cells and in bodily secretions.

2   A range of protein sources in the diet ensures an adequate intake of all the necessary amino acids and the avoidance of deficiency diseases.

3   Extra protein intake is required by those with injury, infection, burns or cancer, as well as at certain times of life, i.e. during pregnancy and when breastfeeding.

4   Protein deficiency is rare in developed countries but common in other parts of the world. Protein and energy deficiencies cause the conditions marasmus and kwashiorkor, which are particularly prevalent in malnourished children.

5   Phenylketonuria is an inherited disorder whereby the amino acid phenylalanine cannot be metabolized. The condition can be treated by diet.

3.6 Minerals

Minerals are only required in small amounts in the diet. Vitamins are also only required in small amounts in the diet and so both groups are sometimes known as **micronutrients.** The most abundant elements in our diet are carbon, hydrogen and oxygen (which are all found in carbohydrates, fats and proteins) and nitrogen (which is present in proteins). However, at least another 16 elements must also be included in the diet. These are the **minerals** and they perform a number of important roles in the body:

1   They form essential *structural* components of cells and tissues; for example, calcium (Ca), phosphorus (P) and magnesium (Mg) compounds are major components of bones and teeth.

2   In their ionized state many of them play an important role in *homeostasis*; for example sodium (Na^+), potassium (K^+), calcium (Ca^{2+}) and chloride (Cl^-) are found in all cells and extracellular fluids.

3   The ions of several minerals (Na^+, K^+, Ca^{2+}) play an essential role in *communication* between cells (for example, in the rapid transfer of information along neurons), and in the transport of small molecules across cell membranes by active transport. For example Ca^{2+} acts as a messenger, transmitting messages within a cell (intracellular) as well as between cells (intercellular) in the brain.

4   Minerals are also *essential components* of many important molecules, including some hormones (for example, iodine (I) is an essential constituent of the thyroid hormones), and many enzymes, which commonly need magnesium or manganese (Mn) to function.

The dietary requirements of minerals are relatively low compared with those of the nutrient macromolecules (**macronutrients**), but some minerals are needed in larger amounts than others. These are known as the major mineral elements, and the minerals required in smaller amounts are the trace elements. The major mineral elements required by the body are shown in Table 3.11 and the trace elements are shown in Table 3.12. You do not need to commit all this information to memory, but do try to remember one or two examples from each Table.

● From Tables 3.11 and 3.12, state which major mineral elements and which trace elements are provided by fruit.

◗ Major mineral elements: potassium, also probably some iron and magnesium (since fruit may also count as 'other vegetables'); trace elements: fruit is not a major source of trace elements, but probably supplies some molybdenum.

Table 3.11 The major mineral elements required by the body. The recommended intakes (RNI) for a woman between 25 and 50 years are listed. The approximate adult body content, functions and common food sources of the minerals are also shown.

Element (symbol)	RNI/g	Body content/g	Functions	Main food sources
calcium (Ca)	0.7	1000	major structural component of bones and teeth; necessary for blood clotting, muscle contraction and conduction of nerve impulses	milk, cheese, bread and flour (if fortified), cereals, green vegetables
chlorine (Cl)	2.5	100	major negative ion (as Cl⁻) in body fluids; present in stomach secretions (as hydrochloric acid, HCl)	salt
iron (Fe)	0.015	4	essential component of haemoglobin in red blood cells	meat and offal, bread and flour, potatoes and other vegetables
magnesium (Mg)	0.3	25	present in bone, inside cells and in body fluids; needed for activity of some enzymes	milk, bread and other cereal products, potatoes and other vegetables
phosphorus (P)	0.55	700	present in bones and teeth; essential for energy storage and transfer by ATP	milk, cheese, bread and cereals, meat and meat products
potassium (K)	3.5	140	main positive ion inside cells; K⁺ also present in extracellular fluids; essential for conduction of nerve impulses, also for the maintenance of ion concentration gradients across cell membranes	widely distributed in vegetables, meat, milk, fruit and fruit juices
sodium (Na)	1.6	100	major positive ion in extracellular fluids; Na⁺ also present inside cells; essential for conduction of nerve impulses and active transport of small molecules across cell membranes (e.g. absorption from gut)	main source is salt (sodium chloride, NaCl) used in food processing, cooking and at the table
sulfur (S)	No value set	150	present in body in proteins	protein-rich foods; meat, fish, eggs, milk, bread, cereals

Table 3.12 Trace elements required by the body. The functions and common food sources of the trace elements are shown.

Element (symbol)	Functions	Main food sources
chromium (Cr)	found in all tissues, may be involved in blood glucose regulation	liver, cereals, beer, yeast
cobalt (Co)	required for formation of red blood cells	liver and other meat
copper (Cu)	component of many enzymes; necessary for haemoglobin formation	green vegetables, fish, liver
iodine (I)	essential constituent of thyroid hormones	milk, seafood, iodized salt
manganese (Mn)	essential component of some enzymes	cereals, pulses, nuts
molybdenum (Mo)	essential component of some enzymes	kidney, cereals, vegetables, fruit
selenium (Se)	essential component of some enzymes; associated with vitamin E activity	cereals, meat, fish
zinc (Zn)	essential component of many enzymes and proteins and in steroid and thyroid hormone activity	meat and meat products; milk and cheese; bread flour and cereal products

A number of other minerals (e.g. silicon and vanadium) are known to be essential in the diet, although their roles have not been established. Yet other minerals, such as fluorine (present as the fluoride ion, F^-, in seafood and some water supplies), have beneficial effects (at appropriate levels), but are not thought to be essential. On the other hand, the body does not readily eliminate minerals so excess intake of many minerals can have toxic effects (see below).

3.6.1 Mineral deficiencies

Because only small amounts of minerals are needed in the diet, and because minerals are abundant in foods, people who eat a varied diet are unlikely to develop mineral deficiency or excess. However, there are exceptions. For example, people who eat food grown in a local region in which there is a mineral deficiency in the soil may have an inadequate intake of that mineral. This is a problem for people in many mountainous areas (particularly the Himalayas and Andes, but also in the Alps and other areas) where iodine is leached from the soil by high rain and snowfall. *Iodine deficiency* has serious consequences; iodine is an essential component of the thyroid hormones (thyroxine and tri-iodothyronine) which are essential for normal growth and for development of the central nervous system. In areas where dietary iodine is lacking, the thyroid hormones are not made in sufficient quantities, and the thyroid enlarges in an attempt to increase production. This is manifested as an enlargement of the throat, known as **goitre**, and is illustrated in Figure 3.14.

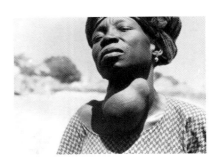

Figure 3.14 The condition of goitre, where the thyroid gland enlarges in an attempt to produce hormones. This it cannot do without an adequate supply of the element iodine.

Nowadays, people in the developed countries are very unlikely to be deficient in iodine, because iodine supplements are added to foods, particularly table salt. However, iodine deficiency is still a serious problem for millions of individuals in the developing world.

Lack of iron is one cause of anaemia. There are several different types of anaemia, which all relate to the inability of the blood to supply cells with oxygen: haemorrhage (blood loss), possibly due to an accident or major surgery is one type of anaemia. Iron-deficiency anaemia is a common mineral deficiency around the world affecting an estimated 10% of the global population. It results in tiredness as well as an increased heart rate, palpitations and rapid breathlessness. Men require 1–2 mg of iron per day and women require 3 mg per day.

● Why do you think women require more iron than men?

● Women lose a significant amount of iron in menstrual blood.

Indeed, iron deficiency is common in women, because of losses during menstruation. Vegetarians are also more likely to experience iron deficiency than are meat-eaters because haem iron (the form of iron in meat, i.e. iron that forms part of the haemoglobin molecule) is more readily absorbed than the iron found in vegetables. Vegetables and fruits contain substances that bind iron compounds and thus reduce iron absorption. An excess of iron can be damaging to the liver, heart and other organs as there is no homeostatic mechanism for disposing of too much iron.

Zinc is necessary for the functioning of a wide variety of enzymes so any deficiency affects most body systems. Processing of food reduces the zinc content and it is suggested that increasingly diets in the developed world leave many children and elderly with mild zinc deficiency (Barasi, 2003). As symptoms include poor appetite and taste acuity, increased vulnerability to infection and slow healing it can be difficult to distinguish from general signs of ageing or malnutrition.

Summary of Section 3.6

1 Minerals are essential micronutrients.

2 Minerals are chemical elements and examples include iron, calcium and sodium.

3 Minerals are essential as structural components of cells and tissues, for homeostasis of ionic balance between body fluids, for communication between cells and as components of other molecules such as haemoglobin, hormones and enzymes.

4 Mineral dietary deficiencies are rare if a balanced diet is consumed; but iron deficiency anaemia is one of the most common whilst the incidence of zinc deficiency appears to be increasing.

3.7 Vitamins

The other dietary micronutrients are the **vitamins**. Vitamins are a chemically diverse group of organic micronutrients that are found in a variety of foods and, like minerals, they cannot (in general) be synthesized by the body. They were named before their detailed chemical structures were known, and so they tend to be referred to by a letter as well as by a chemical name; for example, vitamin D is cholecalciferol and vitamin C is ascorbic acid. Vitamins are divided into two main groups: the fat-soluble vitamins A, D, E and K and the water-soluble vitamins C and B complex. The body can build up stores of fat-soluble vitamins in the liver but the excess of water-soluble vitamins is removed from the body via the urine, so regular intake is necessary. The vitamins, their daily requirements and main food sources are listed in Table 3.13.

Table 3.13 Vitamins essential for human health, their DRVs and main dietary sources (COMA, 1991). NB units are micrograms.

Name	DRV for adults/ μg per day	Main dietary sources
Fat-soluble vitamins		
vitamin A (retinol)	600–700	liver, fish, liver oils, dairy products, also made in the body from β–carotene found in dark green vegetables and carrots
vitamin D (cholecalciferol)	10	margarine, buttermilk, fish-liver oils, oily fish
vitamin E (tocopherols)	3000–4000	plant-seed oils
vitamin K (naphthoquinones)	60–70	green vegetables
Water-soluble vitamins		
vitamin B_1 (thiamin)	1000	nuts, yeast, egg yolk, liver, legumes, meat and cereals
vitamin B_2 (riboflavin)	1000–1300	yeast, green vegetables, milk, liver, eggs, cheese, fish roe
niacin	1200–1700	liver, cheese, yeast, whole cereals, eggs, fish and nuts
vitamin B_6 (pyridoxine)	1400	egg yolk, peas, beans, soya beans, yeast, meat liver
pantothenic acid	7000	many foods
biotin	200	yeast, egg yolk, liver, kidney, tomatoes and intestinal microbes
vitamin B_{12} (cobalamin)	1.5	offal, meat, milk, fortified breakfast cereals
folic acid, folate	200	potatoes, offal, green vegetables, bread, fortified breakfast cereals
vitamin C (ascorbic acid)	4000	green vegetables, fruits, potatoes, blackcurrant syrup, oranges

● Compare Tables 3.10 and 3.13. In the absence of any further information, how could you tell that proteins are macronutrients and vitamins are micronutrients?

● For proteins, the RNI values are in grams per day. For vitamins the DRVs are given in micrograms – a millionth as much.

Vitamins have a variety of roles within the body. Some vitamins and vitamin derivatives are important in *signalling* inside cells. Examples are vitamins A and D, which bind to intracellular receptors and thereby regulate gene transcription and so influence cell function. The activated form of vitamin D promotes transcription of the gene coding for calcium-binding protein. This protein is present on the surface of intestinal epithelial cells and promotes absorption of calcium from the gut (Chapter 4 deals with this in more detail).

Another major role played by some vitamins is that of an **antioxidant**. Vitamins A, C and E and the plant pigment β-carotene (which can be converted in the body into vitamin A) are all antioxidants. Antioxidants play an important protective role, by limiting the action of harmful substances produced by some of the chemical reactions that take place in the body. These harmful substances, known as **free radicals**, are atoms (or groups of atoms) that contain unpaired electrons (that is, electrons that are not currently involved in forming chemical bonds) and so are unstable and highly reactive. They acquire electrons from other molecules that are around them, thus creating another unpaired electron in that molecule and so on, causing a *chain reaction*. This chain reaction can cause considerable damage to living material. Apart from random damage to cells it is hypothesized that free radicals damage DNA molecules.

● What might be the consequence of damaging part of a strand of DNA?

○ Damage to a DNA molecule would affect its ability to replicate faithfully (i.e. the copy would not be pristine: see Section 2.6). If the part of the DNA affected was a coding portion (i.e. a gene) we would describe this as a mutation and it might well result in the cell becoming cancerous.

Antioxidants 'mop up' (i.e. supply electrons to) free radicals, thereby neutralizing them before they can cause too much damage. Free radicals have been implicated in many human diseases and disorders although their exact role has yet to be fully understood. Many pollutants generate free radicals, as does smoking, and it is this that is thought to be their link with diseases such as cancer. You may be pleased to note that other good dietary sources of antioxidants include dark chocolate and red wine.

Vitamin deficiencies, like mineral deficiencies, are now rare in the developed world. However, in some cases, although there may be enough of a particular vitamin in the diet, inadequate amounts of that vitamin may actually be absorbed. For example, vitamin absorption can be reduced if there is too much fibre in the gut, as fibre can bind to some vitamins. There are bacteria in the colon that produce several vitamins. Antibiotic treatment can destroy these bacteria, so this too can reduce the amounts of vitamins that are absorbed. Both a high-fibre diet and antibiotic treatment can thus have serious consequences for people who, due to the quality or quantity of their food, may have a low dietary intake of vitamins.

● Can you suggest some groups that might be at risk of vitamin deficiency?

○ Groups who are considered vulnerable include some older individuals, children and those in hospitals or similar institutions.

3.7.1 Vitamin A

Vitamin A is stored in the liver and adult stores are usually sufficient for 2 years. Vitamin A is also called retinol and is essential in the light-sensitive pigment found in cells in the retina of the eye (Book 2, Chapter 2).

Vitamin A deficiency is one of the top three global public health problems, with a quarter of a million people going blind each year as a result of it. One early symptom of vitamin A deficiency is night blindness. Other symptoms are dry and roughened skin and malformed bones as cell growth and division is disrupted. This disruption also affects other epithelial cell-lined tracts, such as the respiratory, urinary and digestive tracts, which makes them more prone to infection. Vitamin A deficiency in children can slow growth as a metabolite of this vitamin is involved in regulation of genes that mediate growth and development.

● What other role does vitamin A have, and how will health be affected by a deficiency?

◐ It acts as an antioxidant, so deficiency increases damage caused by free radicals within many cell types, and this damage is often a precursor to disease. For example, DNA damage can lead to cancer.

In excess, vitamin A is teratogenic (causes abnormal development) and pregnant women are advised not to eat liver or products made from liver in early pregnancy. Indeed, in some animals such as polar bears so much vitamin A is stored in the liver that eating even a small amount of the liver can be fatal. Overdose of vitamin A can also cause headaches, dry itchy skin and bone and joint pains, although these symptoms can also have a number of other causes.

3.7.2 Vitamin B complex

Vitamin B complex is a group of water-soluble vitamins that promote enzyme activity in a variety of metabolic pathways. Vitamin B deficiency diseases are widespread as these are water-soluble molecules and cannot be stored in significant quantities in the body, so a frequent intake is essential.

Thiamin (vitamin B₁)

Thiamin is important in carbohydrate, alcohol and some amino acid metabolism. The body stores about 30 times the daily requirement of 1 mg, so thiamin deficiencies would be noticed after about a month of a thiamin-free diet. Conversely, a deficiency can be rapidly corrected by thiamin treatment. The deficiency disease, beriberi, is characterized by fatigue and cardiovascular difficulties. Problems associated with maintaining glucose supplies for the nervous system translate into mood changes and progressive neurological degeneration. Beriberi used to be relatively common in communities that subsisted on a diet of polished rice (rice without the husk). Nowadays thiamin deficiency is more often met with in alcoholics who additionally tend to show memory disorder and an inability to coordinate muscular movement. They are described as suffering from Wernicke–Korsakoff syndrome.

Riboflavin (vitamin B₂)

Riboflavin is associated with carbohydrate and protein metabolism, especially in the eyes and skin; deficiency can therefore lead to blurred vision and skin cracking.

Niacin

Niacin can be synthesized from the amino acid tryptophan and is associated with carbohydrate and fat metabolism. It inhibits cholesterol production and aids fat breakdown and has been used to try and reduce cholesterol levels in some patients.

● What is the name of the disorder caused by niacin deficiency and where does it occur?

● Pellagra develops in cases of niacin deficiency in countries where the staple diet is maize because maize is low in tryptophan.

People with pellagra have red skin where it is exposed to sunlight, which may be symptomatic of a general inability to repair skin damage. They may also have anorexia and mental disturbances. The symptoms of pellagra are described in the literature as 'dermatitis, diarrhoea and dementia'.

Vitamin B₆ (pyridoxine)

Vitamin B_6 is associated with fat, glycogen and amino acid metabolism, and the synthesis of non-essential amino acids. Dietary deficiencies of vitamin B_6 are rare, even in the developing world, but deficiencies due to the *availability* of the vitamin can be caused by alcoholism, pregnancy, and taking contraceptive pills or other drugs. Symptoms of deficiency are rather vague and may be ascribed to deficiencies in other vitamins.

Vitamin B₁₂ (cobalamin)

Vitamin B_{12} actually exists as a number of cobalamin compounds, so called because they each contain an atom of cobalt (Co). These large molecules need to be bound to intrinsic factor (a substance made in the stomach) in order to be absorbed from the small intestine (Section 4.3.2). The only dietary source of vitamin B_{12} is animal products, and vegans and vegetarians only avoid vitamin B_{12} deficiency because their plant food is contaminated with trace amounts of it in microbes or faeces-based fertilizers. Vitamin B_{12} is essential for the formation of the fatty myelin sheath that surrounds and protects some neurons, and for DNA synthesis. This latter role means that deficiency immediately leads to problems associated with rapidly dividing cell types such as bone marrow cells. The maturation of red blood cells (erythrocytes) in bone marrow is impaired with vitamin B_{12} deficiency and abnormally large erythrocytes are found in the blood. *Pernicious anaemia* is the most common form of vitamin B_{12}-deficiency anaemia and it is more common in women. Pernicious anaemia is an **autoimmune disease** (one in which the body makes antibodies to its own cells, causing self-cell destruction) in which intrinsic factor is destroyed leading to poor vitamin B_{12} absorption.

Folate

Folate (folic acid) is essential for DNA synthesis.

● Which types of cell will be affected by deficiency of this vitamin?

● Rapidly dividing cell types such as bone marrow cells.

Deficiency of folate leads to another type of anaemia, most commonly seen in pregnant women, called megaloblastic anaemia. This is reversible with folate supplement. It is recommended that women planning pregnancy and those in early pregnancy take folate supplements as these have been shown to reduce the risk of spina bifida (a neural tube defect resulting from the impairment of neural cell division) in the fetus.

Pantothenic acid and biotin

No deficiency diseases have been associated with pantothenic acid and deficiency of biotin is rare. Biotin is important in the synthesis of lipids and glucose and the catabolism of some amino acids. Symptoms of biotin deficiency include anorexia, depression and hallucinations, though these symptoms may have other causes.

3.7.3 Vitamin C

During the 15th century, the need for a diet containing fruit and vegetables to prevent scurvy in sailors was realized (Section 2.11). Sailors who had been at sea for several months without any fresh fruit or vegetables were observed to be losing their hair, have rotten teeth and bleeding gums and very slow healing of wounds. Vitamin C is associated with the formation of a protein called collagen which is found in connective tissue and hair.

Various claims have been made about the ability of vitamin C to stave off colds; however, these claims have not yet been proven in any clinical trials. Vitamin C does, however, enhance the absorption of iron from vegetable sources (known as non-haem iron), so it is important in preventing iron deficiency in vegetarians and vegans.

3.7.4 Vitamin D

● Recall the mechanism that relates vitamin D to bone growth.

● Vitamin D increases transcription of calcium-absorbing protein in the gut epithelium, thereby increasing calcium uptake. Calcium is important for bone formation.

Vitamin D is mostly supplied by metabolic processes that require the exposure of the skin to sunlight; however, it can also be obtained from animal products in the diet.

● Which groups of people are most likely to be at risk of suffering from vitamin D deficiency?

● Children and the elderly, particularly if they are poorly nourished, live in Northern climes and do not get out into the sunlight often. Vitamin D deficiency has also been observed in some cultures that wear clothing draped from head to foot.

Because vitamin D is essential to healthy bone growth, without it children's bones do not become strong enough and their leg bones bow inwards under the weight of their upper bodies, giving them a characteristic 'knock-kneed' posture; this deficiency is known as rickets. In adults the condition is called osteomalacia. These diseases were relatively common in Europe during the 19th century, especially in urban slums. They are now reappearing, most conspicuously in the Asian communities in Northern regions of Europe.

3.7.5 Vitamin E

Vitamin E is a group of eight compounds and is found in cell membranes. Vitamin E acts as an antioxidant. Deficiency of vitamin E is very rare but can be observed in patients with impaired fat absorption.

● Why might vitamin E deficiency be associated with impaired fat absorption?

Because vitamin E is fat soluble and so is absorbed with lipids.

There is some evidence to suggest that vitamin E can help to protect against coronary heart disease, by virtue of its antioxidant properties (see above).

3.7.6 Vitamin K

Vitamin K is synthesized in the large intestine by bacteria in the normal intestinal flora and is absorbed directly. Dietary vitamin K is absorbed from the small intestine with the assistance of bile salts. Vitamin K is required for the synthesis of various blood clotting factors (including the protein *prothrombin*) by the liver and vitamin K deficiency is therefore apparent by a lack of blood clotting. Deficiency can arise if antibiotic treatment kills the intestinal bacteria or they are removed following the use of laxatives. In such cases the body is entirely dependent on an external supply and an adequate diet is important in maintaining this.

Summary of Section 3.7

1   Vitamins are essential organic micronutrients with specific and diverse functions.

2   Vitamins are classified as either fat-soluble or water-soluble. The body can store an excess of fat-soluble vitamins, whereas an excess of most water-soluble vitamins is eliminated from the body in the urine.

3   Some vitamins act as antioxidants, which reduce the effects of the free radicals produced by the body and present in cigarette smoke and chemical pollutants. Free radicals are thought to cause certain diseases and disorders.

3.8 Water

We all know that water is crucial for survival but there is often some confusion about sources of water and their benefit. In addition to drinking pure water we can also hydrate the body by drinking tea, coffee, various juices and milk drinks but not alcohol. Alcohol is a **diuretic**, which means it is a substance that increases the loss of urine from the body. Caffeine is also a diuretic but the amounts found in tea and coffee drinks are insufficient to have a diuretic effect. Levels below 300 mg a day do not have any diuretic effect and, even in the UK, surveys find daily levels well below this value.

We also obtain water from various foodstuffs as shown in Table 3.14.

Individual requirements and intake vary but an average input for an adult might be about a litre of water gained from foodstuffs and a further 1.5 litres drunk during the day. There is also some water gained from metabolic processes, probably less than a quarter of a litre.

● This intake of 2.5–3.0 litres a day is to replace lost water. How do you suppose we lose water?

● The major loss is in the urine and you probably suggested that there would also be loss through the skin as sweat.

Table 3.14 The water content of some foods (as a percentage).

Food	Water
white bread	37
semi-sweet biscuits	2.5
cake	15
cornflakes	3
boiled potatoes	80
potato chips	52
carrots	90
grapes	80
lettuce	95
lentil soup	78
cheddar cheese	36
grilled oily fish	65
cooked meat	60

In fact skin loss occurs over the whole surface of the skin as well as via the sweat glands. The rate of loss through the skin is minimized by the waterproof keratinized layer.

● In what circumstances would this loss become considerable?

● In the case of serious burns to the skin.

Sweat itself is used as part of the regulation of body temperature. Loss of water in sweat increases when it is hot and when exercising. A daily rate of less than 0.5 litres can increase to 2 litres an *hour*. Further water is lost from the surface of the lungs and from the faeces. These are normally fairly steady losses of around 400 ml and 100 ml daily.

● In what circumstances is there a dramatic change in loss of water through the faeces?

● In diarrhoea.

There are many diarrhoeal diseases that spread when people are in over-crowded conditions without a clean water supply and cause death by dehydration.

Urinary output is controlled by the kidney and will be discussed in Book 3. In a dehydrated person it can be as low as 0.5 litres daily and it will be a dark brown colour but 1.5 litres is a more normal output and a light yellow colour reassures that the body is well hydrated.

We have already said that water is essential as a solvent and as a transport system (Chapter 2). You will have noticed that it takes part in metabolic processes itself (e.g. in the breaking down of proteins into their constituent amino acids) and in Book 3 you will learn how it is involved in regulating the ionic balance of body fluids, to ensure homeostasis.

Inappropriate retention of water by tissues causes oedema (swelling) and may be symptomatic of cardiovascular or renal (kidney) problems. Dehydration is detected by *osmoreceptors* in the hypothalamus (on the underside of the brain) and gives rise to a sensation of thirst which will trigger drinking. Obviously it is preferable not to become thirsty though this mild dehydration may not cause any physiological damage. However at even a deficit representing 2% of body weight the nervous system will be affected and symptoms of this level of dehydration may include lack of concentration, irritability, headache and nausea. If dehydration continues more severe symptoms ensue and if untreated the individual eventually falls into a coma and dies.

Summary of Section 3.8

1   Water gained from metabolism, food and by drinking replaces that lost through the skin, faeces, lungs and urine.

2   Water is essential as a solvent, a transport system, as a constituent of metabolic processes and to maintain ionic balance in body fluids.

3   If untreated, dehydration leads to death.

3.9 Conclusions

In this chapter we have tried to show you the roles of the different food groups, and the importance of a balanced diet in maintaining health and withstanding disease. We have hinted that not only are individual nutrients important in their own right, but of equal importance are the interactions between them. Too much or too little of any nutrient can be damaging; of particular concern in modern-day developed societies is the problem of obesity, which results from excessive consumption of any (or all) of the energy-producing foodstuffs. Good nutrition seeks fundamentally to balance TEE and TEI, as well as ensuring adequate levels of micronutrients.

As you read through the chapter you might have been struck by the frequency with which links were made between dietary intake and diseases such as diabetes and cardiovascular disease without there being any details of the mechanisms involved. Although there will be more details in later chapters many of the links are made on epidemiological evidence and we do not yet understand the underlying mechanisms. Sometimes the results of different scientific studies appear contradictory, hence the multiplicity of messages given in the headlines shown in Figure 1.1. However, the value of a balanced and varied diet as the foundation for good health remains incontrovertible.

Questions for Chapter 3

Question 3.1 (LOs 3.1 and 3.4)

If fibre cannot be digested and assimilated, why is it important in the human diet?

Question 3.2 (LOs 3.2, 3.5 and 3.6)

Why is it difficult to assess whether a certain component of the human diet is protective against a disease or disorder?

Question 3.3 (LO 3.3)

(a) What is the body mass index?

(b) Calculate the body mass indexes for Sarah, 1.65 m tall and 55 kg, and Ian, 1.84 m tall and 88 kg. What do the values indicate about the health of these individuals?

(c) Do you estimate yourself to be under- or over-weight, or just right? Calculate your own BMI. What effect does this knowledge have on your perception of your body image?

Question 3.4 (LO 3.6)

Explain, giving examples, why minerals and vitamins can be considered important in communication roles within the human body.

Question 3.5 (LO 3.7)

Your neighbour's normally boisterous 10 year old has been ill and confined to bed for some days. The child has a poor appetite and has been refusing meals but is willing to drink sugary drinks. The neighbour is concerned that this is not healthy and asks for your advice. What would you say?

References

Barasi, M. E. (2003) *Human Nutrition: A Health Perspective*. London: Arnold.

Cockerham, W. C., Hattori, H. and Yamori, Y. (2000) *Social Science and Medicine*, **51**, 115–122.

Committee on Medical Aspects of Food Policy (COMA) (1991) *Nutritional Aspects of Cardiovascular Disease: Report of the Cardiovascular Review Group*. London: HMSO.

Committee on Medical Aspects of Food Policy (COMA) (1994) *Dietary Reference Values for Food, Energy and Nutrients for the UK*. London: HMSO.

Department for Environment, Food and Rural Affairs (DEFRA) (2000) *National Food Survey 2000: annual report on food expenditure, consumption and nutrient intakes*. London: The Stationery Office Ltd.

Department of Health (DoH) (1991) Dietary reference values for food energy and nutrients in the United Kingdom. Report on Health and Social Subjects No. 41. Report of the Panel on Dietary Reference Values of the Committee on Medical Aspects of Food Policy. London: HMSO.

Englyst, H. N., Bingham, S. A., Runswick, S. A. et al. (1998) Dietary fibre (non-starch polysaccharides) in fruits, vegetables and nuts. *Journal of Human Nutrition and Dietetics*, **1**, 247–286.

House of Commons Health Committee (2004) *Obesity. Third Report of Session 2003–04*. London: The Stationery Office Ltd.

Manninen, A. (2004) High protein weight loss diets and purported adverse effects: where is the evidence? *Sports Nutrition Review Journal*, **1**, 45–51.

Office for National Statistics (2003) *Mortality statistics – cause: England and Wales 2002*. London: HMSO.

Pond, C. M. (1998) *The Fats of Life*. Cambridge: Cambridge University Press.

Thatcher, R. (1999) Office for National Statistics, *Population Trends*, **96**, (Summer 1999).

CHAPTER 4

DIGESTION AND ABSORPTION OF NUTRIENTS

Learning Outcomes

After completing this chapter, you should be able to:

4.1 Identify and explain the main functions of the digestive tract and associated organs.

4.2 Describe the different cell types present in the gut and explain their roles in the processing of foods.

4.3 Explain how proteins, carbohydrates and fats are digested in the gut.

4.4 Describe how nutrients are absorbed from the lumen of the gut into the body.

4.5 Explain the physiological processes that give rise to the symptoms seen in a range of disorders of the digestive system.

4.1 Introduction

Growth, development and the maintenance of good health rely upon an adequate supply of nutrients, which must be available to all the cells of the body. The foods we eat are composed of a complex mix of molecules, the majority of which are macromolecules. These are insoluble and too large to be taken up by cells, so must be broken down into smaller, soluble subunits, which can be taken up from the gut into the circulation and then delivered to the different parts of the body. These processes involve the action and interactions of several different organs which are collectively known as the *digestive* or *gastrointestinal system*. In this chapter you will learn about the digestive system and about the physiological processes that are concerned with the digestion and absorption of food.

A number of distinct physiological activities are involved in the assimilation of foods. The processes by which the components of food are broken down in the gut into simpler forms are collectively known as **digestion** and these can be chemical or mechanical. The uptake, into the body, of the products of digestion and of small molecules and ions such as water, mineral salts and vitamins is known as **absorption**. Special **secretions** (i.e. substances made and then exported from cells) are needed to digest foods; important constituents of these secretions include catabolic enzymes that break the chemical bonds linking the components (i.e. subunits) of macromolecules together. The mixing of ingested foods with digestive secretions in the stomach and the propulsion of intestinal contents along the length of the gut are achieved by intestinal movements, which are referred to as gastrointestinal motility. The elimination of faeces (waste matter together with unabsorbed materials) is known as defaecation.

4.2 The digestive system

The gastrointestinal or digestive tract, often simply termed the *gut*, is essentially a very long tube, the shape and dimensions of which vary according to the physiological activities that take place in each particular region. The different parts of the gut are given different names, some of which will probably be familiar to you. The anatomy (structure) of the gut is shown in Figure 4.1. The gut is very long; in an average adult it measures about 7 metres (m) in length. Associated with the gut are a number of other organs that, by producing digestive secretions, play an essential role in digestive processes. These organs, such as the liver and pancreas, are also shown in Figure 4.1.

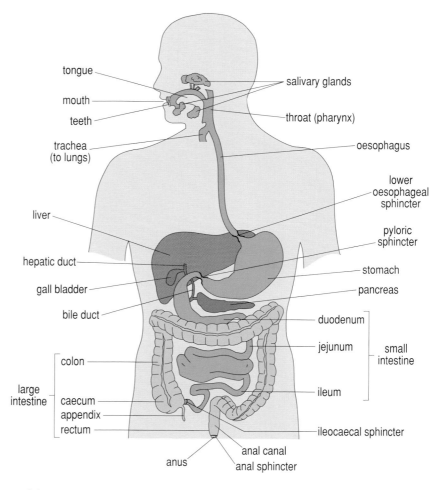

Figure 4.1 Anatomy of the digestive tract (gut) and associated organs.

Foods enter the gut through the mouth, which is involved in the initial processing of food. Chewing and lubrication of each mouthful of food with saliva aids swallowing and eases the passage of the **bolus**, as it is now called, through the throat and, via the **oesophagus**, to the **stomach**. The stomach is a bag-like organ where the first major digestion and mixing processes occur. The partially digested food then passes into the **small intestine** which is the longest part of the gut and is where most digestion and absorption occurs. Some digestive secretions enter the small intestine from the pancreas and the liver, while others are produced by the cells lining the inside of the small intestine itself. The digestion of the dietary macromolecules and the absorption of the products of digestion are largely achieved in the first two parts of the small intestine (called the *duodenum* and *jejunum*); the last part (the *ileum*) provides reserve capacity. Absorption of water and mineral salts, does occur in the small intestine, but mainly occurs in the large intestine.

From the small intestine food passes into the **large intestine**, so called because it is wider than the small intestine. The first part of the large intestine is the *caecum*, which is a pouch-like structure from which the very narrow appendix protrudes. The caecum merges with the major region of the large intestine, known as the *colon*. (Sometimes the term 'colon' is used to describe the entire large intestine.) In the caecum and colon, further absorption of water and mineral salts occurs, concentrating the remains of unabsorbed food and waste products into a semi-solid form called faeces. The colon is also the home of millions of bacteria such as *Lactobacillus*, *Bacteroides*, *E. coli* and *Enterobacter*. These bacteria metabolize soluble fibre into fatty acids, and gases such as hydrogen and methane. The fatty acids can be absorbed and then used by colonic cells as an energy source and the gases are lost as wind.

● Are there any other benefits of having bacterial species living in our colon?

◐ Some of these bacterial species can synthesize vitamins which are absorbed into the body, for example vitamin K as mentioned in Section 3.7.

The last region of the large intestine is the *rectum*, in which faeces remain until they are expelled by passage through the **anus**. These processes are summarized diagrammatically in Figure 4.2.

4.2.1 The structure of the digestive system

Although the shape and dimensions of the gut vary along its length, the organization of the different cell types that make up the gut wall is essentially similar throughout and is shown in Figure 4.3a (overleaf). The three main layers in the gut wall, from the inside outwards, are the *mucosa*, *submucosa* and *muscularis externa*. Each of these layers, in turn, contains several cell types. The *adventitia* (the outer covering of any organ is called adventitia) does not form an integral part of the gut wall.

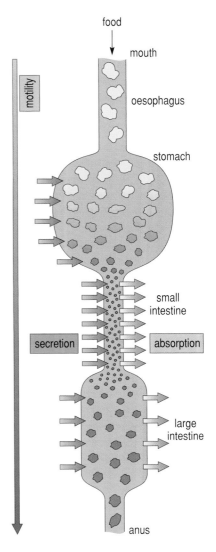

Figure 4.2   Diagram illustrating the processes occurring in the different parts of the gut.

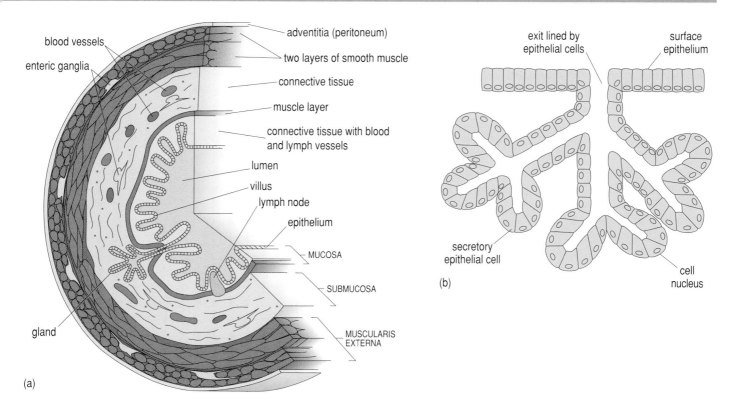

Figure 4.3 (a) Diagram of a cross-section through the gut wall showing the three main layers and the different cell types present. (b) A gland, formed by invagination (infolding) of mucosal epithelium.

Mucosa

The mucosa is the layer of cells lining the lumen (inside) of the gut. In fact, the inside of the gut is continuous with the outside of the body (the two meeting at the mouth and the anus) and, like the skin, it is a major interface between the internal environment and the outside world. The properties of the epithelium of most parts of the gut, however, are rather different from those of the skin. In some areas such as the mouth, oesophagus and anus, where some physical protection is needed, the epithelium is several layers thick and is something like that of the skin. In most parts of the gut, however, the epithelium is only a single cell thick, with the **apical** membrane of these cells exposed to the lumen of the gut and the **basal** membrane opposite, against the submucosal cells. (*Apical* relates to the apex of a pyramid and *basal* relates to the base of a pyramid.) The epithelial cells are specialized to perform digestive or absorptive roles, for example the epithelial cells in the small intestine have small hair-like projections called **microvilli** on their apical surface. As you will see, digestive functions are carried out both by secretions (including enzymes) from specialized epithelial cells and also by enzymes that are *not* secreted but are an integral part of the epithelial cell membrane. In the stomach and intestines, the epithelium is frequently invaginated (i.e. folded inwards) to form glands, as illustrated in Figure 4.3b. Glands consist of groups of secretory epithelial cells; different types of gland are found in different regions of the gut. These glands do not have ducts.

There is an extremely rapid turnover of epithelial cells in the gut. In the small intestine some 17 billion epithelial cells are shed into the lumen and replaced each day, the entire epithelium being renewed every five days. The rapid and continual turnover of the epithelium makes this tissue very sensitive to agents that inhibit cell division, such as radiation and the drugs used in chemotherapy for the treatment of cancer.

If you look again at Figure 4.3a, you will see that on the basal membrane of the epithelium is a layer of connective tissue, which is richly supplied with blood vessels and also with lymph vessels. It is here that the absorbed nutrients enter the bloodstream or, in the case of fats, the lymphatic system. Blood passes from the intestinal vessels directly to the liver, via a blood vessel known as the hepatic portal vein.

Despite the protective nature of epithelium, and the bactericidal (bacteria-killing) action of stomach secretions, some **pathogens** (potentially damaging small organisms such as microbes that cause disease) do gain entry into the body from the gut lumen. As protection against these pathogens, the connective tissue immediately below the epithelium is well supplied with cells from the immune system (discussed in detail in Book 3, Chapter 4).

Submucosa

The next major tissue layer is called the submucosa (see Figure 4.3a). This is a loose matrix (mixture) of connective tissue in which lie blood and lymph vessels, and a large number of neuron cell bodies grouped together as **ganglia**. These neuron cell bodies are part of the **enteric** (relating to the intestine) **nervous system**. The enteric neurons extend to the mucosa, where they influence both the production of digestive secretions by the epithelial cells and also the state of dilation of the mucosal blood vessels.

Muscularis externa

The muscularis externa is a thick layer of **smooth muscle**. In contrast to **skeletal muscle** it contracts spontaneously, in a rhythmic fashion, without any input from nerves, although its activity is constantly being modulated by the **autonomic nervous system** and by hormones. The autonomic nervous system controls the automatic functions within our body that we do not consciously control, i.e. involuntary actions, and the **somatic nervous system** controls the voluntary actions, such as moving of limbs; this will be covered in some depth in Chapter 1 of Book 2.

In fact the muscularis externa consists, in almost all parts of the gut, of two separate muscle layers that lie at right angles to each other. The outer muscle layer is longitudinal, that is it runs lengthways along the gut and the inner muscle layer fibres encircle the wall of the tube. Successive contraction and relaxation of these muscle layers results in **peristalsis**, waves of movement that propel the bolus through the gut, as illustrated schematically in Figure 4.4 (overleaf). Peristalsis is controlled by the action of another group of enteric neurons that lie in ganglia between the outer smooth muscle layers (Figure 4.3a).

Although most gut movements (and other gastrointestinal processes) occur involuntarily, there are two parts of the gut where strong, short-lived voluntary

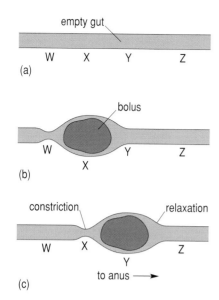

Figure 4.4 Peristalsis. The smooth muscle cells of the muscularis externa contract behind a bolus of food, but relax ahead of it, propelling the bolus along the length of the gut: (a) muscle layers relaxed; (b) contraction at W and relaxation at X followed by (c) contraction at X and relaxation at Y results in movement of the bolus towards the anus.

control is needed: (a) the throat and upper oesophagus, which are involved in swallowing; and (b) the external anal **sphincter**, which relaxes during defaecation. A sphincter is a constriction in a tubular organ, such as the gut, surrounded by a ring of either smooth or skeletal muscle; relaxation and contraction of this muscle controls the opening and closing of the sphincter. In both these regions of the digestive tract, skeletal muscle takes the place of smooth muscle. Skeletal muscle is under voluntary control.

● Can you suggest whether the anal sphincter and pyloric sphincter are controlled by the autonomic or somatic nervous systems? (You may like to look back at Figure 4.1 to remind yourself of the locations of these sphincters.)

○ The anal sphincter is under voluntary control so therefore controlled by the somatic nervous system and the pyloric sphincter is not voluntarily controlled so is therefore under the autonomic nervous system control.

Adventitia (outer covering)

The outer covering of the gut (the adventitia) is loose fibrous tissue around the oesophagus but becomes a serous (watery-fluid-producing) membrane called the **peritoneum** around the remainder of the gut. The peritoneum is a closed sac, which acts as a physical barrier to the local spread of infection, such as when the appendix becomes infected and inflamed in appendicitis. In severe cases of appendicitis the appendix can rupture and the peritoneum can become infected (peritonitis), which can prove fatal. Surgical removal of an inflamed appendix should prevent peritonitis occurring as the spread of infection is stopped.

Summary of Section 4.2

1   The digestive system is responsible for the processing and absorption of nutrients from food and the absorption of water.

2   The gut is a tube-like organ that can be divided into regions where different stages in the processing and absorption of foods occur.

3   The main physiological processes performed by the gut are:
   • digestion of food by production of digestive secretions and churning;
   • absorption of the products of digestion as well as mineral salts, vitamins and water;
   • motility, which allows movement of contents by peristalsis;
   • elimination of undigested and unabsorbed gut contents;
   • defence against pathogens.

4   The gut wall consists of several different cell types and components:
   • epithelial cells, specialized for secretion or absorption;
   • smooth muscle cells, responsible for motility;
   • enteric neurons, essential for the coordination of gut functions;
   • blood and lymph vessels, allowing transport of absorbed nutrients to the rest of the body;
   • immune system cells, providing defence against ingested pathogens.

4.3 Passage of food along the gut

Now you have a general picture of the organization of the gut, we can turn to how the digestive system actually processes foods. Perhaps the easiest and most logical way to describe this is to follow what happens when we eat a meal. First, however, we should reconsider the molecular nature of the foods we eat.

4.3.1 The human diet

● Can you remember what the six main nutrients in the human diet are?

● Proteins, carbohydrates, lipids (fats), vitamins, mineral salts and water.

Most of the foods we consume consist of insoluble macromolecules, large molecules that are too big to cross cell membranes by diffusion. These macromolecules need to be broken down into their smaller constituents as shown in Table 4.1 before they can pass through the epithelial cells of the mucosa into the blood and lymph vessels to be transported around the body.

Table 4.1   The macromolecule components of the human diet and their small molecule components.

Macromolecule	Small molecule components
protein	amino acids
carbohydrate	monosaccharides (sugars)
lipids/fats – not strictly macromolecules but aggregates	fatty acids and glycerol

Carbohydrates, proteins and fats are the major components of our diet. The task of the gut is to break down these large molecules into their simpler and smaller components. Most of these smaller molecules are soluble and with the aid of specialized molecules and processes (to be described shortly), can then cross the epithelial cell membranes into the blood and lymph systems and so be transported around and assimilated into the body. Vitamins, minerals and water do not need to be broken down into smaller components to be absorbed from the gut.

Before it reaches the main part of the digestive system, material that is to be digested must be bitten, chewed and swallowed. The process of digestion, then, actually begins with ingestion via the mouth.

4.3.2 Mouth

Although human diets are varied, most consist of at least a proportion of very bulky material such as vegetables, and tough material such as meat. For food to be digested it must be in contact with the digestive secretions that act on it, so the bulky food material must first be broken down into small pieces; this process serves to increase the surface area of the food, thereby making it more accessible to the digestive secretions.

The initial processing of the food is performed in the mouth, and involves the actions of the tongue, teeth, jaws and secretions produced by the salivary glands. The arrangement of these structures is shown in Figure 4.5.

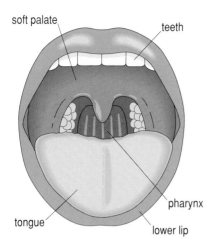

Figure 4.5 The structures visible in a wide open mouth.

Humans (and most other mammals) have two sets of teeth in a lifetime. The first set of teeth is known as **milk teeth** and usually erupts (breaks through the gums) at between seven months and two years of age, although there is considerable variation in this. There are 20 milk teeth, which are lost gradually during childhood (usually between seven and 13 years of age) and are replaced with what are optimistically called **permanent teeth**. The full complement of permanent teeth in the adult varies between 28 and 32, some individuals having wisdom teeth, which are the last permanent teeth to erupt, at the back of the mouth. The incisors (front teeth) cut off pieces of food; canines, premolars, and molars chew and grind the food, mixing it with saliva (Figure 4.6).

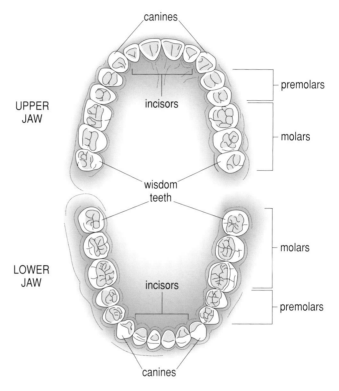

Figure 4.6 Diagram showing a complete set of permanent teeth, including the wisdom teeth.

The structure of a tooth is shown in Figure 4.7. The part of the tooth that protrudes into the mouth is known as the **crown**; the part that fits in the jaw is the **root**. The crown is covered by a substance called **enamel**. Enamel is the hardest material in the body and, if well looked after, is very resistant to corrosion by acids and enzymes. It consists of a very strong protein, similar to keratin, in which large, dense crystals of calcium salts (calcium carbonate and calcium phosphate) and other minerals (e.g. sodium, magnesium and potassium salts) are embedded.

Within the enamel is the *dentine*, which forms the main part of the tooth and has a similar composition to bone. The innermost part of the tooth is known as the *pulp*, and is composed of connective tissue and is supplied with blood vessels,

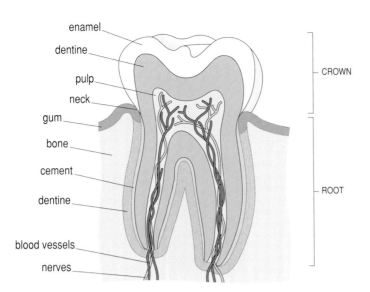

enamel
dentine
pulp
neck
gum
bone
cement
dentine
blood vessels
nerves

CROWN

ROOT

Figure 4.7   Diagram of a vertical section through a tooth.

nerves and lymph vessels. The tooth is held in place by peridontal ligaments, consisting of tightly packed collagen fibres, and by a substance called *cement*, which is secreted by the cells lining the tooth socket.

The development of teeth begins when the embryo is six weeks old, and continues during fetal development and childhood. The formation of healthy teeth is dependent upon an adequate supply of minerals, particularly calcium and phosphate, and also vitamin D (which plays an important role in calcium absorption, as you will see later) and parathyroid hormone (which stimulates the formation of the active form of vitamin D).

Teeth are a dynamic part of the body; mineral salts are constantly being absorbed from the teeth into the bloodstream and at the same time, new material is deposited. Evidence suggests that this turnover of minerals occurs mainly in the dentine and cement, and that little occurs in the enamel. For this reason the enamel is particularly vulnerable if damaged (Box 4.1).

Box 4.1 Dental caries

The main damage that occurs to teeth in the western world is the formation of **caries** (cavities) due to decay. The moist film of saliva, food and bacteria covering the teeth is called **plaque** and sugars present in plaque serve as an ideal source of nutrients for the *Streptococcus mutans* (*S. mutans*) and other bacteria that normally live there. These plaque bacteria produce an acid called lactic acid and **proteolytic enzymes** (enzymes that break down proteins). Over a period of time, the acid gradually dissolves the calcium salts in the enamel producing a cavity. This then allows rapid digestion of the enamel protein remaining, by the bacterial proteolytic enzymes (and also by proteolytic enzymes present in saliva). Although the enamel presents an extremely resistant barrier to this process, once decay has penetrated this layer, the underlying dentine is much more vulnerable and more easily dissolved. The problem of caries is almost entirely due to our consumption of sugary foods and acidic carbonated drinks and the frequency with which we eat foods (snack) between main meals.

Prevention of dental caries by thorough and regular toothbrushing is emphasized by dentists and children should be encouraged to brush their teeth from a very early age.

The movements of the teeth, **mastication** or chewing, are controlled by the activity of the jaw muscles. During chewing, the food is broken into smaller pieces and mixed with saliva, produced by a number of glands collectively known as the **salivary glands**. Acute inflammation of the salivary glands by the mumps virus is called mumps and this was far more prevalent before vaccination of preschool children against this viral disease.

As we start to eat, sensory nerves in the mouth are activated in response to the stimuli of taste and pressure. These activate neurons in the brain which, in turn, activate the neurons innervating (supplying) the salivary glands, and so stimulate the secretion of saliva. **Salivation** (the secretion of saliva from salivary glands) is also stimulated in response to the sight, taste and smell of food and even by the thought of food.

About 1.5 litres of saliva are produced each day and saliva consists of a watery solution of mineral salts and several other components. The two main components are an enzyme called **salivary amylase**, which begins the digestion of the carbohydrate starch breaking it down into the disaccharide maltose and short polysaccharide chains, and **mucus**, which is a glycoprotein and acts as a lubricant.

● What is a glycoprotein composed of?

○ A glycoprotein is composed of both protein and carbohydrate (Section 3.3).

Saliva also contains small amounts of **lysozyme** (an antibacterial, proteolytic enzyme) and antibodies, and it is slightly acidic. It plays an important part in oral hygiene – not only does it wash food particles and bacteria away from the teeth into the gut, but the lysozyme, antibodies and weak acid attack the bacteria in the mouth.

The tongue is a large muscular structure at the floor of the mouth. It plays an important role in mastication of food as it moves food around the mouth and then to the back of the mouth in a bolus to initiate swallowing. The tongue (as well as the lips and cheeks) is also crucial in speech as it manipulates the sounds from the vocal cords into recognizable words. The top surface of the tongue consists of numerous papillae (small projections) which contain nerve endings of sensory neurons; these are called taste buds (Figure 4.8). The papillae are of four different types:

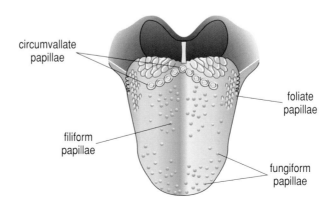

Figure 4.8 Location of the papillae of the tongue.

- circumvallate and foliate papillae are the largest and are arranged at the base of the tongue; they detect the bitter taste;

- fungiform papillae are more numerous and are situated at the tip and edges of the tongue; they detect sweet and salty/sour tastes;

- filiform papillae are the smallest of the papillae and are located towards the centre of the tongue; their role is mechanical rather than taste detection.

The categorization of taste into sweet, sour, salty and bitter is an over-simplification. A combination of these tastes and the texture, viscosity and even temperature of food all contribute to our experience and enjoyment of food. The sense of smell is closely linked to taste and this greatly enhances our taste experience – just think how bland food tastes when you have a stuffy nose! (The taste buds are covered in more detail in Book 2, Chapter 2.)

The sense of taste triggers salivation and the secretion of **gastric** (relating to the stomach) juice in the stomach. It can also be protective, for example when foul tasting food is eaten the gagging or vomiting reflex can be triggered so expelling the possibly toxic food. The senses of smell and taste often decrease with age, the loss of taste being associated with the loss of taste buds. This is an important consideration when planning meals for older people, as the flavours may need to be stronger than would normally be used to enable them to taste the food. It also helps explain why some older people can start to have symptoms of malnutrition as their taste wanes and they lose interest in eating.

Summary of Section 4.3.2

1   The initial processing of food is carried out in the mouth, by the teeth, which break the food into small pieces and mix it with saliva.

2   An adult will have between 28 and 32 permanent teeth, protected by hard enamel.

3   Saliva has an antibacterial action and contains salivary amylase, which begins carbohydrate digestion.

4   The tongue plays a crucial role in mastication, taste and speech.

4.3.3 The oesophagus

Swallowing is a complex reflex which is partly involuntary and partly under voluntary control. When food is forced to the back of the mouth by the tongue, pressure receptors in the throat are activated. These relay signals to part of the brain called the swallowing centre (in the brainstem; Book 2, Chapter 1), which in turn activates nerves supplying the muscles of the throat, larynx, oesophagus, diaphragm and intercostal (breathing) muscles. Swallowing requires the coordinated activity of all these muscle groups, so that breathing is interrupted to allow food to pass into the oesophagus and not into the trachea and lungs. In fact in the pharynx (part of the throat where the oesophagus and trachea join), the larynx (organ of voice production) rises up to meet with the epiglottis to close off the trachea to any swallowed food (Figure 4.9, overleaf). This involuntary response prevents the blockage of the trachea or choking and if the swallowing reflex is impaired the stomach contents can be regurgitated and inhaled.

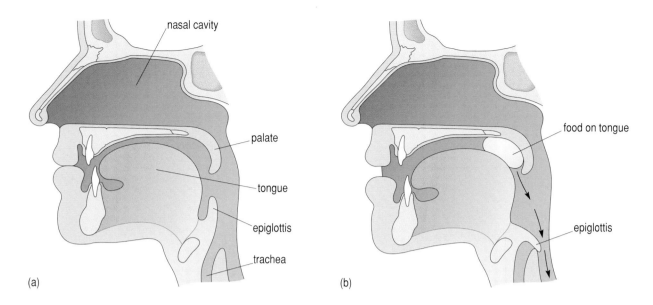

Figure 4.9 A section of the face and neck showing the position of structures (a) before and (b) during swallowing.

Food passes down the oesophagus to the stomach as a result of a wave of peristalsis.

● Which types of cell are involved in peristalsis?

◉ Peristalsis occurs because of the contraction and relaxation of the outer layers of smooth muscle cells in the gut wall and is controlled by enteric neurons.

This wave of peristalsis passes along the length of the oesophagus in about 8–10 seconds and is triggered by the presence of a bolus of food. The lower oesophageal sphincter (a ring of thickened smooth muscle where the oesophagus meets the stomach; Figure 4.1), which is normally closed to protect the oesophagus from the acidic contents of the stomach, then relaxes, thereby allowing food to enter the stomach. The sphincter and the upper stomach muscles relax in a process known as *receptive relaxation*, which is controlled by enteric neurons.

The lower oesophageal sphincter is a weak sphincter and can open inappropriately in some people resulting in reflux (return) of the stomach contents, known in its mild form as *heartburn*. Too much reflux of stomach contents back into the oesophagus can cause inflammation (swelling) of the lower end of the oesophagus. This can cause significant discomfort when swallowing and can be relieved by antacids (acid-neutralizing compounds) and local anaesthetics (pain killers). In more severe cases of reflux, drugs which stimulate oesophageal motility can be prescribed as this should help to keep the oesophagus empty. Obese people with reflux problems are advised to elevate their bedhead during sleep.

Oesophageal cancer is the ninth most common cancer and it occurs more frequently in males than females. The presence of an oesophageal tumour is often not noticed until trouble is experienced swallowing. Tumours in the oesophagus lead to death by oesophageal obstruction if not treated sufficiently early.

Summary of Section 4.3.3

1 A peristaltic wave passes the bolus of food down the oesophagus, through the lower oesophageal sphincter and into the stomach.

2 Reflux of stomach contents can result in heartburn.

4.3.4 The stomach

The stomach is a muscular bag-like organ in which food is partially digested and stored until it is transferred to the small intestine. The stomach undergoes great changes in size, varying in volume from 50 ml when empty, to 1500 ml (1.5 litres) after a large meal, i.e. increasing its size 30 times. The processing of food in the stomach is achieved by mixing the contents with digestive secretions produced by specialized epithelial cells of the gastric mucosa. The mixing occurs as a result of waves of contraction of the smooth muscle of the stomach wall.

The presence of food in the stomach triggers the secretion of digestive juices. However, observation of the timing of such secretion shows that rather than responding to the presence of food in the stomach, we normally start to respond before the food has even got into the stomach. In effect, we anticipate its arrival.

● What is the biological advantage of such anticipation?

○ The food arrives in a stomach that is immediately able to start the digestive process. It avoids time delays. This might be of advantage at times when food is in short supply and the body is nutrient-deficient.

● What could be the disadvantage of this anticipatory response?

○ The production of gastric juice would be an unnecessary expenditure of energy if no food were to arrive in the stomach. (Also the acidic nature of the gastric secretions could be harmful to the stomach cell wall.)

The mucosal epithelium of the stomach contains many glands formed by invagination.

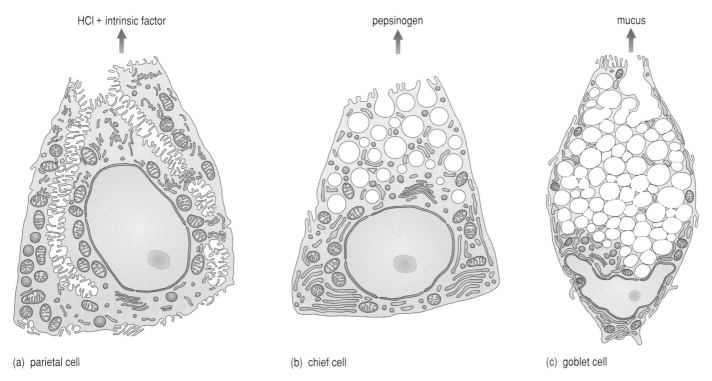

(a) parietal cell   (b) chief cell   (c) goblet cell

Figure 4.10 Cells from stomach gastric glands (a) parietal cells, (b) chief cells and (c) goblet cells.

Cells in these glands (Figure 4.10) are specialized to produce a number of different gastric secretions, all with a different role:

- **Hydrochloric acid (HCl)**, from the parietal cells, helps to dissolve the lumps of food entering the stomach. HCl is a strong acid which is almost completely dissociated (separated) in solution into hydrogen (H^+) and chloride (Cl^-) ions. The high concentration of hydrogen ions makes the gastric secretions very acidic. The degree of the acidity is measured as a pH value (see Box 4.2). The pH of the gastric secretions is between 1.5 and 3.0. The hydrogen ions help to disrupt (denature) the physical structure of some of the macro-molecules in food, especially proteins, and allow the enzymes easier access. Some enzymes such as salivary amylase are also denatured in the acid conditions. The acidity of the gastric secretions also kills most ingested microbes.

- **Intrinsic factor**, from the parietal cells, is a protein and is necessary for vitamin B_{12} absorption in the small intestine.

● What disease can occur if the stomach does not release intrinsic factor?

◐ Pernicious anaemia (see Section 3.7.2).

- **Pepsinogen**, from the chief cells, is converted into the active enzyme **pepsin** by HCl, and pepsin begins the breakdown of proteins into polypeptide chains and peptides. Unlike most enzymes which are active at physiological pH (6–8) pepsin is active at pH 1.5–3.0. Between 10% and 20% of total protein digestion occurs in the stomach.

- Mucus, from the goblet cells, acts as a lubricant and prevents injury to the stomach by the corrosive hydrochloric acid. This provides a less acid *microenvironment* (i.e. local environment), with a pH of between 5 and 6 which is substantially less acidic than other areas of the lumen.

Another important molecule is also produced by the gastric mucosa, the hormone **gastrin**. Gastrin is secreted into the *blood vessels* of the mucosa rather than into the stomach from specialized epithelial cells. It reaches and activates other epithelial cells of the gut, including nearby acid-secreting epithelial cells and also epithelial cells secreting digestive molecules further along the gastrointestinal tract.

Box 4.2 The pH scale

The pH scale runs from 1 to 14 with pH 7 on the scale being neutral, 1–6 on the scale being acidic and 8–14 on the scale being alkaline. Pure water has a pH of 7.0; physiological systems usually have a pH of between 6 and 8. The extracellular fluids of the body (interstitial fluid, lymph and blood) have a slightly alkaline pH with a normal range of between 7.35 and 7.45, while intracellular fluids have a slightly lower pH of between 7.0 and 7.2. Stomach contents are very unusual, in having a pH of between 1.5 and 3.0. A very small change in the pH of body fluids can have severe implications as cells are tuned to operate within very narrow pH ranges.

The food arriving in the stomach is usually still rather bulky and consists mainly of small lumps. Contractions of the smooth muscle of the stomach wall mix the stomach contents with HCl; this dissolves the lumps, forming a thick, soup-like mixture called **chyme**, made up of liquid and small particles of food. Chyme allows easier access to digestive enzymes, which would not effectively penetrate lumps of food.

Gastritis is a common condition occurring when there is too much gastric juice and too little mucus to protect the mucosal cell layer, which becomes inflamed and destroyed by the HCl. The most severe gastritis is acute haemorrhagic gastritis when the epithelial cells are destroyed and blood is lost into the stomach. The causes of gastritis are varied and include; regular and excessive alcohol consumption, food poisoning, heavy smoking and prolonged use of aspirin and other **non-steroidal anti-inflammatory drugs (NSAIDs)**.

Stomach cancer is the sixth most common cancer in the UK. The growths destroy the normal mucosal cell layer resulting in reduced HCl secretion and subsequent pH increase in the stomach. Intrinsic factor release is also compromised and one of the first symptoms a patient with stomach cancer may experience could be weakness and fatigue due to pernicious anaemia. Other initial symptoms include: indigestion or a burning sensation (heartburn); discomfort or pain in the abdomen; nausea and vomiting; diarrhoea or constipation; bloating of the stomach after meals; loss of appetite; bleeding, including either vomiting blood or blood in the faeces. None of the symptoms are exclusive to stomach cancer.

The acidic environment in the stomach has been blamed as the cause of the common condition of peptic ulcers. There are a range of symptoms associated with peptic ulcers and they can often occur with the ingestion of food. They include: nausea, heartburn, discomfort and gastric pain. Ulcers are formed by erosion of the gut epithelium which can, in severe cases, extend to deeper layers of the gut wall. The underlying causes are unclear but if a healthy mucosa is not maintained, HCl gains access to the epithelium causing initial cell damage leading to ulceration. The predisposing factors are thought to be:

- reduced blood supply, possibly due to smoking or stress;

- altered mucus secretion, possibly due to prolonged aspirin use amongst other factors (see below);

- reduced epithelial cell replacement, possibly due to raised steroid hormone levels (either as a natural response to stress or when used as drugs);

- infection by a bacterium, *Helicobacter pylori* (*H. pylori*). This bacterium is found in 67% of patients with gastric ulcer and 90% of patients with duodenal ulcer. It appears that the bacterium resists destruction by acid in the stomach by adhering to the mucosa, beneath the protective layer of mucus and that it produces toxins that cause damage to epithelial cells.

Treatment of peptic ulcers used to be with antacids such as magnesium trisilicate and aluminium hydroxide which reduce the acidity and pepsin activity in the stomach. However, treatment now is often in three stages:

(i) Acidity reduction. The parietal cells release H^+ ions (also called protons) into the stomach. The protons cross the cell membrane via a membrane protein that is therefore called a protein pump. Certain drugs target the release of protons by blocking the action of the pumps either directly or indirectly; examples include cimetidine, ranitidine and omeprazole.

(ii) *H. pylori* eradication. This bacterial infection can be treated with the antibiotics amoxycillin and clarithromycin. Eradication of *H. pylori* is very important in preventing ulcer recurrence.

(iii) NSAIDS avoidance. This large drug group is used to treat minor pain by suppressing prostaglandin release. One group of prostaglandins are substances released by damaged cells that are associated with the sensation of pain and with inflammation (swelling and redness). However, prostaglandin E2 is a member of another prostaglandin family and is released by the stomach epithelial cells to help with the secretion of mucus; a decrease in mucus secretion makes the epithelial cells more vulnerable to attack by HCl. It is for this reason that most NSAIDs should be avoided in peptic ulceration treatment if possible.

As well as pathogenic microbes, another threat from food is the possible ingestion of toxic substances. Exposure to such agents is a normal part of everyday life and reflexes have evolved that eliminate the potentially hazardous substances as rapidly as possible. The first of these to come into operation after ingestion is vomiting. In addition to removing the noxious agent from the gut, it is thought that vomiting may have an additional adaptive benefit, for the nausea that usually accompanies vomiting can lead to learning to avoid further ingestion of the same substance.

Like swallowing, vomiting is a complex reflex, which requires coordinated responses by a variety of muscles. It is regulated by a centre in the brainstem called the vomiting centre. The vomiting reflex can be triggered by a number of different stimuli, the commonest being excessive distension of the stomach and small intestine and activation of *chemoreceptors* (receptors that respond to stimuli of a chemical nature) in the gut by harmful chemicals or toxins. Other stimuli, originating outside the gut, can also activate the vomiting centre.

Examples of such stimuli include increased pressure in the skull (e.g. concussion), movements of the head that do not match with other sensory inputs (motion or travel sickness) and chemical stimuli that affect the vomiting centre. An example of this could be intravenous treatment with cytotoxic (cell-poisoning) drugs for cancer therapy although simply knowing that the drugs are going to be administered can trigger vomiting in some patients, an example of learning that psychologists call a 'conditioned response'.

Anti-emetics are drugs used to prevent or diminish vomiting and they are prescribed according to the cause of vomiting.

Summary of Section 4.3.4

1   In the stomach, muscular activity mixes the food with gastric secretions to make chyme.

2   The pH in the stomach is very acidic at pH 1.5–3.0 and this denatures proteins including the enzyme salivary amylase, activates pepsin from pepsinogen and has an antimicrobial function.

3   Mucus protects the epithelial cells of the stomach from the action of hydrochloric acid.

4   The stomach has three types of epithelial cell which produce gastric secretions: parietal cells secrete HCl and intrinsic factor, chief cells secrete pepsinogen and goblet cells secrete mucus.

5   Peptic ulcers form if the epithelial cell layer is eroded by acid; this condition is often associated with *H. pylori* infection.

6   The vomiting reflex can remove noxious substances from the stomach although it can also be triggered in some other circumstances such as in motion-sickness.

4.3.5 The small intestine and its associated glands

After being processed in the stomach, chyme enters the small intestine in controlled bursts, not in a continuous flow. At the junction between the stomach and the first part of the small intestine is an area of thickened smooth muscle, similar to that at the base of the oesophagus. This is the *pyloric sphincter* (Figure 4.1). Waves of contraction of the stomach muscle reach the sphincter, causing it to close. Between contractions, the smooth muscle relaxes, opening the sphincter. The rate of muscle contraction, then, is important in the regulation of the rate at which chyme passes from the stomach to the small intestine. The time it takes a meal to pass through the stomach is also dependent on the nature of the foods eaten, but is usually between two and six hours.

The small intestine is essentially a long tube, with a diameter of about 4 cm and a length of about 5 m, which is divided into (naming from the stomach) the duodenum, jejunum and ileum (Figure 4.1). The main roles of the small intestine are the completion of enzymatic digestion of macromolecules and the absorption of the small molecule products. The surface area of the small intestine is greatly increased by the presence of numerous finger-like projections called **villi** (singular, villus, see Figure 4.11). There are about 20–40 villi per square millimetre (mm²) of mucosa, and each villus extends about 0.5–1.5 mm into the lumen. A further increase in surface area is provided by tiny projections from the surface of individual epithelial cells. These structures are the microvilli and they form what, for obvious reasons, is called the **brush border** of the cell (Figure 4.11, inset). The combined increase in the surface area of the epithelium resulting from these specializations is about 600-fold, making the surface area of the human small intestine approximately 300 square metres – about the same area as that of a tennis court.

Figure 4.11 Villi, regular finger-shaped projections of the mucosal layer, which increase the inner surface area of the gut; note the microvilli on the epithelial cells (inset) which increase the surface area still further.

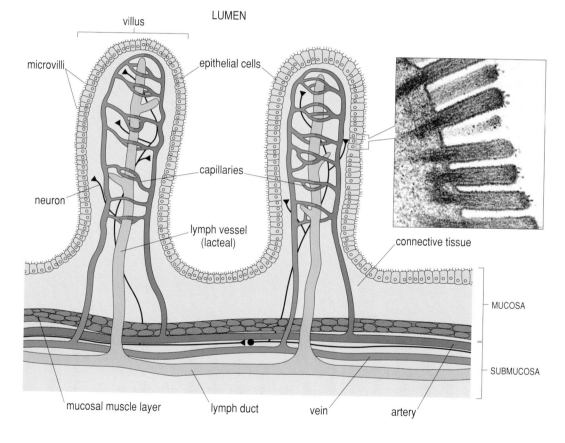

- What advantage is conferred by having this huge surface area?
- The larger surface area allows a greater area for the absorption of nutrients into the blood system.

- Looking at Figure 4.1 can you suggest another adaptation of the small intestine that creates a larger surface area?
- The small intestine is greatly folded.

You have seen how, in the stomach, the complex mix of macromolecules that we eat is digested both physically and chemically to a soup-like chyme.

● Name the two main macromolecular constituents of our diet that have been partially digested by the time they leave the stomach and their products. Which chemicals are required to effect this digestion?

○ (i) Proteins have been denatured and partially broken down into peptide fragments by the action of hydrochloric acid and pepsin in the stomach.

(ii) The carbohydrate starch has been partially broken down into the disaccharide maltose and short-chain polysaccharides by the action of salivary amylase.

The digestive processes of the small intestine are concerned with breaking down these molecules into yet smaller components.

Look again at Figure 4.1 and you will see that there is a duct (a small tube) which is connected to the duodenum almost immediately after the junction of the stomach and small intestine. This duct is the route by which two other digestive secretions enter the gut lumen. These secretions are produced by the liver and the pancreas. Both these organs perform several different functions, and are not just involved in digestion. This is an example of the complex *interdependence* of body systems; they do not operate in isolation.

The pancreas

The pancreas is a long gland lying adjacent to the duodenum, behind the stomach (Figure 4.1). The pancreas produces exocrine secretions; these are fluids that are secreted via ducts, onto the surface of an epithelial tissue. (Sweat glands of the skin are another example of exocrine glands.) Most of the pancreas consists of exocrine tissue which is organized as groups of epithelial cells clustered around a central duct. Secretions from the cells pass into the duct, which then joins to other, larger ducts that finally convey the secretions, together with those from the liver, via the sphincter of Oddi (Figure 4.12), into the duodenum.

Lying within this exocrine tissue of the pancreas are groups of endocrine (hormone-releasing) cells known as **islets of Langerhans** (Figure 4.12). The islet cells secrete several hormones into the bloodstream, including two that play an important role in homeostasis (the maintenance of the internal environment within narrow limits, see Section 2.4) of blood glucose levels. The homeostatic maintenance of blood glucose levels will be discussed in more detail in Book 2, Section 3.7, but for now you need to know that blood glucose levels are maintained at approximately 4–6 millimoles per litre of blood to prevent damage to surrounding cells.

Hormones often control homeostatic processes and blood glucose level is maintained by the hormones **insulin** and **glucagon**. Insulin is released from the β cells in the islets of Langerhans in the pancreas in response to high blood glucose levels (usually following a meal) and glucagon is released from the α cells of the islets of Langerhans in response to low blood glucose levels. The action of insulin results in glucose being taken up by liver and muscle cells and being converted into glycogen. Glucagon activity reverses this process by initiating the breakdown of glycogen in muscle and liver cells and its subsequent release into the bloodstream. The deficiency or impairment of insulin activity is known as **diabetes mellitus** (commonly simplified to **diabetes**) and it results in raised blood glucose levels. Excess glucose is excreted in the urine (glucosuria) and the person becomes very thirsty. Diabetes will be discussed in more detail in Book 2, Chapter 3.

Figure 4.12 Diagram showing the organization of the endocrine and exocrine cells of the pancreas (not to scale).

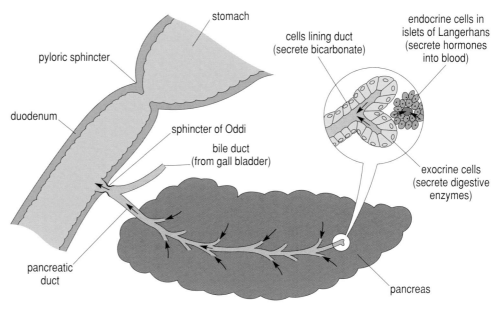

What, then, is the nature of the pancreatic products involved in digestion? The exocrine glands of the pancreas produce a variety of digestive enzymes, which will be described shortly. In addition, they produce bicarbonate ions (also known as hydrogen carbonate ions), HCO_3^-. These ions neutralize the acid in the chyme by combining with the H^+ ions to form carbonic acid which is a very weak acid.

● What will happen to the pH of chyme on leaving the stomach and combining with the pancreatic secretions?

◉ The pH will increase from the range of 1.5–3.0. (In fact it increases to pH 6–7, i.e. becomes neutral.)

● Why is it important that the pH becomes neutral?

◉ Most enzymes are inactivated and denatured by acid solutions, so before the digestive enzymes of the small intestine can set to work to further break down the partially digested proteins and carbohydrates present in the chyme, the H^+ ions must be quickly neutralized.

Along with HCO_3^- ions, the pancreas produces a number of digestive enzymes. Like pepsin in the stomach, the digestive enzymes produced by the pancreas are almost all manufactured as precursor molecules which are converted into the active enzyme in the gut lumen. Pancreatic enzymes are activated by the action of another enzyme, situated in the membrane of the intestinal epithelial cells (unlike the enzymes we have discussed so far, all of which are free in the gut lumen). This enzyme is called *enterokinase* and it acts on *trypsinogen* to produce the proteolytic enzyme **trypsin**. Trypsin then activates other digestive enzymes in a similar way, i.e. by splitting off peptide fragments from the precursors. This sequence of enzyme activation is illustrated in Figure 4.13. Some other pancreatic enzymes are not produced as precursors, but are only fully activated when they reach the gut lumen, where they encounter an appropriate molecular/ionic environment.

If the proteolytic pancreatic enzymes are activated before leaving the pancreas, cell damage occurs and this is known as *pancreatitis*. The severity of the pancreatitis relates directly to the amount of tissue destroyed and severe forms can cause cell death and haemorrhage. The causes of pancreatitis are not fully defined although gallstones and alcoholism are predisposing factors.

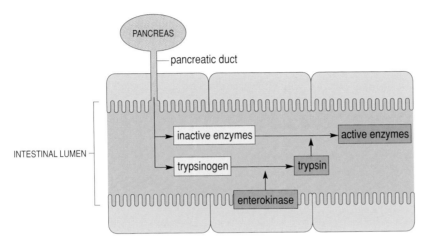

Figure 4.13   The activation of pancreatic enzyme precursors in the small intestine.

As shown in Table 4.2, the pancreas produces a rich mix of enzymes. These include: a number of proteolytic enzymes; **pancreatic amylase**, which breaks down polysaccharides; **lipase**, which breaks down lipids; and also nucleic acid-digesting enzymes (nucleases).

Table 4.2   The pancreatic enzymes, their substrates and actions.

Enzyme	Substrate	Action
trypsin, chymotrypsin, elastase	proteins	break peptide bonds in proteins to form peptide fragments
carboxypeptidase	proteins and peptides	removes terminal amino acid from carboxyl end of chain
pancreatic amylase	polysaccharides	splits polysaccharides into disaccharides and short chains of glucose units (dextrins)
lipase	lipids	splits two fatty acids from each triacylglycerol molecule, forming free fatty acids and monoacylglycerols
nucleases (ribonuclease, deoxyribonuclease)	nucleic acids (RNA and DNA)	split nucleic acids

The liver

The liver is the largest gland in the body, lying just beneath and slightly behind the stomach (Figure 4.1). The liver is a complex organ and it is involved in digestive processes and a number of important processes that are summarized in Box 4.3.

The liver synthesizes and secretes **bile** – an exocrine secretion – into the duodenum.

● What are exocrine secretions?

● Exocrine secretions are fluids that are secreted via ducts onto the surface of an epithelial tissue.

Bile is an aqueous mixture of substances including bicarbonate ions (HCO_3^-), phospholipids, cholesterol and cholesterol-derived molecules known as bile salts. Also present in bile are waste products of the various processing reactions of the liver (see Box 4.3).

● What function would the bicarbonate ions serve?

● They neutralize the acidic chyme.

Bile salts aid fat digestion by emulsifying fats (this is covered in detail in the next section). Bile is secreted from the liver into the duodenum through a tube called the hepatic duct. Between meals the bile is stored in a small bag-like structure, the **gall bladder** (see Figure 4.1). The gall bladder is not an essential organ and can be removed without ill-effect, as long as the hepatic duct is left intact. Sometimes the salts and cholesterol of bile can form deposits known as gallstones in the gall bladder. The presence of gallstones can be unknown until they move and become stuck in the bile duct when severe pain is felt.

Summary of Section 4.3.5

1   The chyme passes through the pyloric sphincter into the small intestine and is mixed with digestive juices produced by the pancreas and liver. It is in the small intestine that most digestion and absorption occurs.

2   The walls of the small intestine have villi and the apical surface of the epithelial cells has microvilli; these structures greatly increase the surface area of the small intestine for absorption.

3   The pancreas produces digestive enzymes as inactive precursors which are activated in the lumen of the gut by trypsin and bicarbonate (hydrogen carbonate) ions (HCO_3^-) to neutralize the acidic chyme.

4   The liver also produces HCO_3^-, additionally it secretes bile which emulsifies fat.

5   The liver is the largest gland in the body with a range of functions including digestive, homeostasis, metabolic, excretory and storage.

Box 4.3 The liver

The liver has several functions in addition to its role in digestive processes.

It has an important homeostatic role in relation to regulation of blood glucose levels.

● What is this role?

● The liver *responds* to the presence of the two hormones, insulin and glucagon. High levels of insulin in the bloodstream stimulate the liver cells (hepatocytes) to remove glucose from the blood and convert it into glycogen which is then stored. High levels of circulating glucagon stimulate hepatocytes to break down the stored glycogen, thereby releasing glucose back into the bloodstream.

The liver stores other substances including fat-soluble vitamins; A, D, E, K as well as the minerals iron and copper. Some water-soluble vitamins are also stored, e.g. riboflavin, niacin, pyridoxine, folic acid and Vitamin B_{12}. The liver also converts amino acids into fatty acids for storage following a meal, but during fasting it converts fatty acids into ketones which can be used as an energy source.

There are other interconversions involving amino acids, lipids and carbohydrates, notably cholesterol is synthesized and released into the bloodstream under certain conditions, whilst at other times it is converted into bile salts. New amino acids are synthesized from amino acid breakdown, and any nitrogenous waste from the process is converted into urea and excreted in urine.

The liver is involved in the synthesis of blood plasma proteins (e.g. globulins, albumin, lipoproteins) and clotting factors from amino acid precursors. Whilst in its excretory role the liver destroys old red blood cells, the major product being bilirubin from the haemoglobin, which is then excreted in bile. It also plays a crucial role in protecting our body against drugs and other noxious substances (such as microbial toxins) by detoxifying them and excreting the products. The liver also metabolizes ethanol (alcohol).

Because the liver is involved in so many metabolic processes, it is the main heat-producing organ of the body.

There are some substances that we ingest that the liver removes from the bloodstream and takes into storage but then, having no mechanism for their disposal, can itself be damaged as the amount in storage increases. These include some manufactured chemicals such as certain pesticides, but also substances that are desirable in low dosages.

● Can you give an example of a substance in the latter category?

● Yes, iron was noted to be in this category (Section 3.6).

Many of the drugs that are modified (for excretion) in the liver can cause damage to the liver during this process, the extent of the damage depending on the size of the dose. An overdose of paracetamol can induce severe liver damage, which can prove fatal. The number of paracetamol tablets that can kill varies between individuals with some requiring only a very few tablets and others requiring significantly more. This illustrates how our genetic make-up influences our responses to drugs; the study of this area is known as 'pharmacogenetics'. Early symptoms of paracetamol overdose are minimal and it is only after 2 or 3 days that jaundice with liver and kidney failure can cause death. Other substances toxic to the liver include cytotoxic drugs, anabolic steroids and alcohol. These substances can cause cirrhosis of the liver, which is a progressive disease of the liver characterized by damage to liver cells often leading to jaundice. Jaundice is not a liver disease in itself but is a sign of abnormal bilirubin metabolism in which unconjugated bilirubin increases to a dangerous level in the blood. Unconjugated bilirubin is not joined to its protein carrier. This leads to yellow colouration of the skin and in severe cases can cause fits and brain damage. Hepatitis is liver cell damage or necrosis (cell death) and can be due to viral infections, toxic substances (as just mentioned including drugs and alcohol) and circulatory problems. Viral infections are the most common form of **acute** (short-lasting and relatively severe) hepatitis and include types A, B and C. Viral type A is the mildest infection; it is spread by the faecal–oral route. Types B and C cause more severe infections and are spread via blood and blood products; type C is prevalent among intravenous drug users. **Chronic** (long-lasting) hepatitis persists for more than 6 months and can be associated with type B and C viruses and some unpredictable drug reactions.

4.3.6 Digestion and absorption of nutrients in the small intestine

At this stage in the passage of a meal through the gut some digestion has taken place but we still have some large insoluble molecules that form the major part of the human diet and that need to be broken down into smaller, soluble molecules. In this section, you will see how these macromolecules are further broken down and the digestion products are actually absorbed into the body, via the intestinal epithelium. This necessitates crossing the epithelial cell membrane.

● The cell membrane forms an effective barrier between the internal and external environments of the cell. Bearing in mind the composition of the cell membrane (Section 2.5.1), which type of molecule would be likely to enter the intestinal epithelial cell membrane most easily?

● The hydrophobic fats will have the easiest job diffusing across the epithelial cell membrane because of the hydrophobic nature of the membrane itself. (Another substance that can freely cross cell membranes is alcohol, which explains why it is readily absorbed into the bloodstream, even from in the stomach – with the result that its effects are felt very rapidly!)

Proteins and amino acids

Proteins entering the duodenum from the stomach are broken down further into peptide fragments by the pancreatic enzymes trypsin and chymotrypsin (Table 4.2). These proteolytic enzymes cleave peptide bonds after specific amino acids, resulting in a range of peptide fragments of different length. The peptide fragments are too large to be absorbed across the epithelial cells into the blood, so are broken down further into free amino acids by two enzymes: carboxypeptidase, which is secreted by the pancreas, and aminopeptidase, which is located in the brush border of the intestinal epithelial cells (Table 4.3). Carboxypeptidase releases amino acids from one end of the peptide chain; aminopeptidase releases amino acids from the other end of the chain.

The end-products of protein digestion, then, are free amino acids. If food is chewed thoroughly, 98% of ingested protein can be broken down to amino acids and absorbed, and only 2% will be excreted in the faeces.

Table 4.3 Enzymes of the intestinal epithelium.

Enzyme	Substrate	Action
aminopeptidase	proteins and peptides	removes terminal amino acid from amino end of chain
dextrinase	dextrins (short chains of glucose units)	splits dextrins into glucose units
lactase	lactose (milk sugar)	splits lactose into glucose and galactose
sucrase	sucrose (table sugar)	splits sucrose into glucose and fructose
maltase	maltose (a disaccharide produced by the action of amylase on starch)	splits maltose into two glucose units

● What is the nature of the free amino acids that inhibits their passage into the epithelial cells?

● They are charged hydrophilic molecules (Table 3.8).

● How might they cross the membrane?

● Free amino acids cross the epithelial cell membrane by active transport, i.e. requiring energy (ATP) to power the process. (See Figure 2.10.)

The amino acids bind to a protein molecule spanning the width of the membrane, known as a *transporter*. This amino acid transporter pumps amino acids and sodium ions together across the epithelial cell membrane into the epithelial cell, a process known as cotransport. The absorbed amino acids then leave the epithelial cells via the basal and lateral (side) areas of the cell membrane by one of several possible processes, to enter the capillaries present in the villi.

Carbohydrates and monosaccharides

You have already seen that digestion of starch begins in the mouth and continues for a short time in the stomach, until the salivary amylase is inactivated by acid. Pancreatic amylase then continues the digestion of starch into molecules containing different numbers of glucose molecules. (You do not have to remember the names of these molecules but starch is digested to the disaccharide *maltose*, the trisaccharide *maltotriose* and the short polysaccharide *α-dextrin* by pancreatic amylase.) Maltose and maltotriose are broken down into glucose molecules by the enzyme *maltase*, present on the brush border. Dextrins are broken down by an enzyme called *dextrinase*, also located on the brush border (see Table 4.3).

The disaccharide *lactose*, is the only sugar present in milk and this is split into one molecule of glucose and one of galactose by the enzyme *lactase*. Lactase is an essential enzyme in new-born babies, since their only source of sugars is the lactose in milk.

● Why is it essential that there is a source of sugar in breast milk?

● It is essential to supply glucose to brain cells as these are still developing and cannot use other energy sources.

During adolescence, however, some individuals gradually lose lactase from the brush border, until it is completely absent. The absence of lactase is termed *alactasia*. Since disaccharides cannot be absorbed, any deficiency in the enzymes that convert disaccharides into monosaccharides will result in an accumulation of that disaccharide in the gut lumen. So, consumption of milk by adults who have no lactase in the gut results in accumulation of lactose in the gut. This leads to an influx of fluid from the intestinal blood capillaries via the interstitial fluids into the small intestine due to the osmotic effect (see Box 4.4) and an expansion in the population of gut bacteria that use lactose as a food source.

● What clinical symptoms would you expect to see?

● The clinical symptoms are severe watery diarrhoea, abdominal pain and distension or bloating.

This extreme reaction of lactose intolerance is often triggered by even small amounts of milk. Milk products in which lactose is converted into other forms, such as the lactic acid in yoghurt, may be tolerated by individuals with alactasia.

Lactose intolerance should not be confused with galactosaemia, a severe inherited disorder in which the metabolism of galactose is inhibited. This enzyme deficiency is further down the metabolic pathway from lactose and afflicted babies fail to thrive on milk. Vomiting and diarrhoea occur on consumption of milk. Galactosaemia is treated by simply excluding galactose from the diet, although this can be difficult for some parents to achieve.

● Can people with galactosaemia drink milk?

○ No, because the sugar in milk is the disaccharide lactose and this is broken down by lactase to glucose and galactose.

Normally all carbohydrates are broken down to monosaccharides which can be carried into the epithelial cells. Transport proteins are involved in the absorption of monosaccharides, but (as you may have suspected) they are not the same proteins as those that carry amino acids into these cells. Glucose and galactose are very similar in structure and are both transported across the apical epithelial cell membrane by the same family of glucose transporter proteins. These glucose transporters use energy to transport sodium ions into the epithelial cell with the monosaccharide. It is thought that fructose also crosses the epithelial cell membranes by using transporter proteins but not using energy. This can be achieved because fructose is transported down its concentration gradient, i.e. to areas of lower concentration. This is known as passive transport or passive diffusion.

Once absorbed into the epithelial cells, monosaccharides leave via the basal and lateral cell membranes by facilitated diffusion, as illustrated in Figure 4.14. This figure shows that glucose is pumped from a low concentration in the lumen of the small intestine to a higher concentration in the epithelial cell itself. This means that glucose is being transported against its concentration gradient and explains why energy is needed to make this occur. However, glucose leaves the epithelial cell via a glucose carrier to a less concentrated area in the blood and so energy is not required and so the transport is by facilitated diffusion.

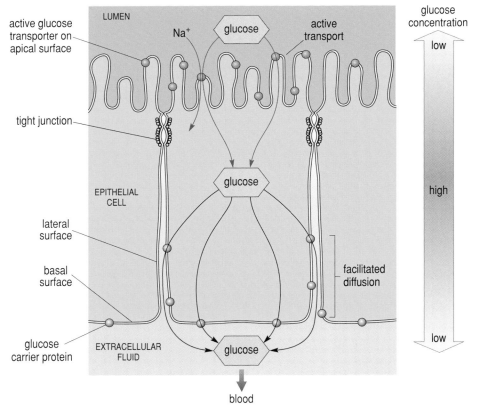

Figure 4.14 The transport of glucose through an intestinal epithelial cell.

Box 4.4 Osmolarity and osmotic pressure

The concentration of H_2O in pure water is 100%. Water in the body contains dissolved solutes, including potassium, sodium and chloride ions, and sugars such as glucose. Therefore the concentration of water in body fluid is reduced by the presence of solutes. The greater the solute concentration, the lower the concentration of water. Adding water to a sample of body fluid will increase the concentration of water; adding more solute, e.g. glucose, will reduce the concentration of water. The concentration of water in body fluid depends on how many 'particles' of solute there are per unit mass of water. One molecule of glucose is one particle; one sodium ion is a particle too; the total concentration of solute particles in water is known as its **osmolarity**, hence we measure concentrations in moles (i.e. number of particles). If body fluid contains a high concentration of particles and therefore low water concentration, it is said to have a high osmolarity. Imagine a person is dehydrated and feeling thirsty. The blood will have a high osmolarity and therefore a low water content, and in such a case, the blood is described as having a high osmotic pressure. The latter term derives from the response of cell membranes to exposure to solutions. Cell membranes are semipermeable, that is, they allow passage of water and small solute particles, but large molecules such as proteins cannot cross. If cells are bathed in body fluid of high osmolarity, then the water inside the cell will exit through the cell membrane until both body fluid and cells have the same osmolarity. The term osmotic pressure refers to the pressure that would have to be applied to the solution to prevent the net flow of water into the solution, in this case, the body fluid. The movement of water across a cell membrane is termed **osmosis**. Cellophane provides a useful model for a semipermeable cell membrane. If a small amount of a concentrated solution of sucrose, e.g. treacle, is placed in a cellophane bag and this is immersed in a large beaker full of water, then the bag will gradually fill with water, until the sugar concentration is the same on both sides of the cellophane membrane.

Lipids and fatty acids

Lipids or fats are not as simply digested as proteins and carbohydrates as they are not soluble in the aqueous solutions found in the gut lumen. Because fats do not dissolve in water, when mixed with an aqueous solution they separate out and form a layer on top of the liquid, in a similar manner to oil spilt at sea. Perhaps a more relevant example, since we are considering digestion, would be the layer of fat that forms on the top of a stewed meat dish. This property of fats means that the way in which they are digested is very different from the ways in which proteins and carbohydrates are broken down.

Lipids associate together as globules or large droplets in aqueous solutions and the digestive enzyme lipase (from the pancreas) only has access to the outer molecules of the globule. If lipid digestion occurred in this manner it would be a very slow and inefficient process. Therefore the first thing that needs to happen to these fat droplets is that they are dispersed into much smaller droplets and this occurs by the action of bile salts in a process known as **emulsification**. This is similar to what happens when washing up liquid is added to greasy water. Emulsification greatly increases the surface area of fat droplets accessible to lipase (see Figure 4.15) which acts on triacylglycerols by splitting off two of the three fatty acid units, leaving a *mono*acylglycerol and two free fatty acids.

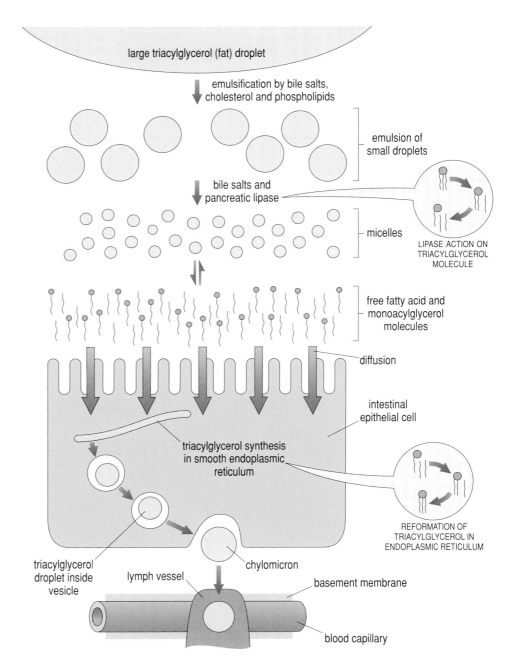

Figure 4.15 Diagram summarizing the emulsification, digestion and absorption of fats.

These products of lipid digestion are, like the lipid substrate itself, almost insoluble in water, so we would expect them to also associate into large droplets making their absorption from the aqueous lumen very slow. However, this process is accelerated due to the formation of tiny structures (much smaller than the droplets in an emulsion) called **micelles**. These are aggregates of bile salts, phospholipids, fats and the products of lipase action – fatty acids and monoacylglycerol molecules (Figure 4.15). The formation of micelles is a dynamic process, i.e. they are continually breaking down and reforming. This means that they provide a reservoir of fatty acids and monoacylglycerols which can move into solution in the lumen and are able to diffuse into the brush border of the intestinal epithelium (see below). Fat-soluble vitamins, such as vitamin D, are also transferred to the brush border in the micelles.

Fatty acids and monoacylglycerols are able to diffuse from the lumen across the cell membrane into the epithelial cells. The only limiting factor to this process would be if the concentration of fatty acids inside the cell was much greater than that outside the cell, in the gut lumen (as is the case for glucose).

Once they enter the epithelial cells, the fatty acids and monoacylglycerols are converted back into triacylglycerols (within the smooth endoplasmic reticulum), and these once again aggregate, together with phospholipids, cholesterol and fat-soluble vitamins, into small droplets known as **chylomicrons** (Figure 4.15). This *sequestration* into chylomicrons ensures that the concentration of *free* fatty acids inside the cell is kept low, so that more are able to enter the cell by diffusion following their concentration gradient. The chylomicrons accumulate inside vesicles which bud off from the smooth endoplasmic reticulum and are transported (via the Golgi apparatus) to the basal side of the epithelial cell. Here the vesicles fuse with the cell membrane and expel the chylomicrons into the interstitial fluid (i.e. the fluid filling the spaces between cells) by exocytosis. Chylomicrons cannot enter the bloodstream directly, since they cannot pass across the basement membrane (a layer of glycoprotein) which surrounds blood vessels. Instead the chylomicrons enter the lymph vessels, via the large pores in the vessel walls; from here, they are transported into the bloodstream.

Minerals and vitamins

As you know from the last chapter, sodium is an essential element, present in its ionic form as Na^+ ions. On average, most of us consume some 5–8 g (grams) of sodium each day and an additional 20–30 g are added to the gut in the various secretions that enter it.

- You have already learnt about many of the secretions entering the gut. Can you list them?

- Saliva, gastric secretions, bile and pancreatic secretions.

Most of the sodium that enters the gut is absorbed in the small intestine. Sodium ions are predominantly absorbed by active transport, together with amino acids and monosaccharides as described in Figure 4.16 (overleaf).

Figure 4.16 Diagram showing the major routes by which amino acids, monosaccharides and sodium ions are absorbed into the intestinal epithelium. Amino acids and monosaccharides are absorbed by active transport, coupled with sodium ions. The sodium pump removes Na^+ out of these cells into the interstitial space, and generates the gradient of Na^+ concentration which is required to drive the cotransport of amino acids and mono-saccharides. Water is absorbed by osmosis, through the spaces between the epithelial cells, when the Na^+ concentration in the interstitial space is greater than that in the lumen. When levels of Na^+ in the lumen are higher than in the interstitial space, Na^+ is absorbed by diffusion, also through these spaces.

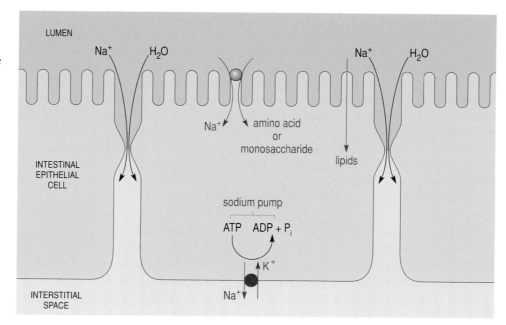

Other mineral ions, such as potassium and magnesium are absorbed by active transport without difficulty but calcium is poorly absorbed from the gut. In fact, about 87% of the daily intake of calcium is not absorbed, but excreted in the faeces.

● Which vitamin must be present to enhance the absorption of calcium?

◗ Vitamin D is involved in aiding calcium absorption.

It does this by stimulating the formation of the calcium transporter protein in the epithelial cell membranes.

Iron is interesting because it can be absorbed in several different ways. Iron in the diet occurs in two forms: in the organic molecule haem (present in meat and fish) and in iron salts (from eggs and plants). Whereas haem iron is relatively easily absorbed, only 10–15% of ingested iron salts enter the bloodstream, a fact that clearly has implications for vegetarians. Iron salts need to be converted into a form that can be absorbed in the gut lumen and this process is greatly enhanced by vitamin C. However, in contrast to the case of vitamin D and calcium, vitamin C must be present in the gut at the same time as the iron to be effective in this way. Other dietary components, such as calcium, soya protein and some constituents of vegetables, actually inhibit iron absorption, as already mentioned in Chapter 3.

Most water-soluble vitamins are small molecules and are absorbed either by passive diffusion or by facilitated diffusion. Vitamin B_{12}, however, is a large, charged molecule and so cannot be absorbed directly.

● What factor is required for vitamin B_{12} absorption?

◗ Intrinsic factor is required.

Vitamin B_{12} binds to intrinsic factor from the parietal cells of the stomach and later, in the ileum the resulting complex binds to specific receptors on the surface of epithelial cells. This binding can *only* take place if vitamin B_{12} is bound to intrinsic factor. So the presence of the intrinsic factor is thus essential for absorption of the vitamin.

Water

In addition to intake in the form of drink, water also forms a significant component of the foods we eat. In fact, a vast amount of fluid enters the digestive tract. Each day, in addition to ingesting up to about two litres of water, the secretions of the digestive system add a further seven litres of water to the lumen of the gut.

The sources of the water that enters the digestive tract per day are shown in Figure 4.17. Almost all this water is absorbed in the small intestine; approximately 80–90% of the remaining half litre is absorbed in the large intestine, leaving only about one-tenth of a litre which passes out in the faeces.

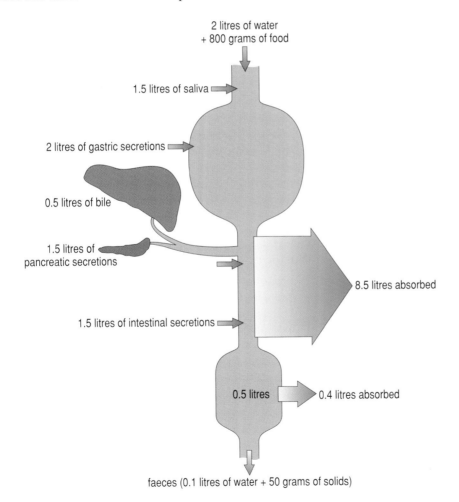

Figure 4.17 Diagram showing the sources of water that enters the digestive tract per day, and the regions from which water leaves.

How is all this water absorbed? The answer to this is that there are very small pores between the epithelial cells in the small intestine (see Figure 4.16). Water crosses into the interstitial space between the epithelial cells by osmosis. Most of the water is absorbed by this *paracellular* route; as shown in Figure 4.16, some diffusion of ions (e.g. Na^+) occurs here too. However, some water movement occurs by a *transcellular route*, i.e. across the epithelial cell membrane, into the cytosol and then out of the cell into the interstitial space (not shown in Figure 4.16).

The absorption of water, then, is inextricably tied up with that of salts, and is dependent upon the concentration difference between the interstitial space and the gut lumen.

● The chyme is very concentrated when it first reaches the lumen of the duodenum. Will water move into the interstitial space under these circumstances?

● No, not if the solute concentration in the lumen is greater than that in the interstitial space. In fact, water leaves the interstitial space and enters the lumen, by osmosis, under these circumstances.

As nutrients and ions are absorbed, however, the chyme becomes more dilute, and water is then absorbed. It should be added that absorption is an ever-changing process, the type and extent of absorption of the various nutrients in different gut regions depending on the conditions that prevail there at any particular time.

Chyme takes 4–6 hours to pass through the small intestine. It then enters the large intestine, slowly, through the ileocaecal sphincter (see Figure 4.1). This sphincter prevents the chyme from passing back into the small intestine when the large intestine is distended.

Summary of Section 4.3.6

1   Proteins are finally broken down in the small intestine into amino acids by the combined action of trypsin, chymotrypsin, carboxypeptidase and aminopeptidase.

2   Carbohydrates are broken down into monosaccharides by enzymes on the brush border of the epithelial cells.

3   Amino acids and monosaccharides are absorbed into epithelial cells by Na^+-coupled active transport using specific transport proteins.

4   Absence of lactase, which breaks down the disaccharide lactose found in milk, results in lactose intolerance in adults.

5   Lipids are emulsified by the action of bile salts and lipases break them down into free fatty acids and glycerol molecules.

6   Lipids diffuse into the epithelial cells and into the lymph vessels.

7   Vitamin D aids calcium absorption into the epithelial cells.

8   The mineral iron is taken into the diet in two different ways. Haem iron (found in meat) is easily absorbed, whereas iron salts (found in eggs and plants) are more difficult to absorb and require the presence of vitamin C.

9   Water is absorbed mainly from the small intestine via paracellular and transcellular routes by the process of osmosis.

4.3.7 The large intestine

The large intestine starts at the caecum and terminates at the anus as illustrated in Figure 4.1. Like the small intestine, it is a tube-like organ, but with a larger diameter – about 6 cm – and is about 1.5 m long.

From the preceding section, it should be clear that most digestion and absorption occur in the small intestine. In fact, a considerable proportion of the small intestine serves as reserve capacity as far as the absorption of amino acids, mono-saccharides and fatty acids is concerned. The bulk of absorption that occurs in the large intestine is of water and salts, and only about 4% of digested material is absorbed in this last part of the digestive tract.

The large intestine plays a special role in the absorption of vitamins. This is of importance if dietary intake of vitamins is low. The large intestine is populated by bacteria, which synthesize several vitamins, including vitamin B_{12} (although, as mentioned above, some is ingested in food), vitamin K, thiamin (vitamin B_1) and riboflavin (vitamin B_2). The production and absorption of vitamin K, which plays a role in blood clotting, is of particular importance, since levels of this vitamin in food are usually inadequate.

● What effect does taking antibiotics have on the absorption of these vitamins?

○ Treatment with antibiotics can destroy these intestinal bacteria and can therefore sometimes cause vitamin deficiency in individuals whose vitamin intake is low and who therefore depend on vitamin formation and absorption in the large intestine.

Some foods, such as beans, contain a large proportion of fibre (non-digestible carbohydrates) that cannot be digested by human digestive enzymes.

● How is this fibre broken down?

○ Bacteria in the colon break down the soluble NSP and resistant starch components of fibre resulting in the daily production of about 0.4–0.7 litres of gas – predominantly nitrogen and carbon dioxide, but also small amounts of hydrogen, methane and hydrogen sulfide; this is why consumption of certain foods produces a lot of wind!

The consumption of fibre has other important consequences; the rate of movement of faeces along and out of the large intestine is related to their bulk. Stools containing a lot of solid material are larger, and their passage along the large intestine is accelerated. This is because distension of the gut is one of the important stimuli that result in the activation of the smooth muscle of the gut wall.

● Can you think of any benefits of having a high proportion of fibre in your diet?

○ High-fibre diets are thought to be protective against colon cancer, heart disease and diabetes; there is also a lower incidence of diverticular disease with diets high in fibre (Section 3.3.2).

The gut contents move relatively slowly, taking between 12 and 24 hours, depending on diet, to pass from the ileocaecal sphincter to the rectum. Peristalsis occurs less frequently in the large intestine than in the small intestine (about twice an hour) and the strong wave of peristalsis is known as mass movement. Mass movement is often triggered by entry of food into the stomach and this response is known as the *gastrocolic reflex*.

Chyme entering the large intestine contains, for the most part, secretions from the lower part of the small intestine, wastes from the liver, undigested material and fibre. The absorption of water in the large intestine results in the formation of the faeces (or stools). These are normally composed of about two parts of water and one part of solid material, the latter dead bacteria, fibre and undigested material, small amounts of bile pigments, cholesterol, fatty acids and mucus secreted from the epithelial cells of the large intestine.

Mass movement of the colon contents into the rectum stimulates defaecation. The nerve endings (receptors) are triggered by stretch and infants will defaecate by a reflex action. The reflex action can be overridden and this control is learnt usually in the second or third year of life. The acquired voluntary control means that defaecation can be inhibited by the brain until it is convenient to go to the toilet. Repeated suppression of the urge to defaecate may lead to constipation.

There is one other part of the large intestine, which we should mention, and that is the appendix. If you look again at Figure 4.1, you will see that the appendix is situated just after the junction between the small intestine and caecum. The role of the appendix is not clear, but it contains abundant lymphoid tissue, particularly in children. This lymphoid tissue is not present at birth, but appears progressively during the first 10 years of life, after which it gradually disappears; the normal adult appendix contains only traces of lymphoid tissue. Although the presence of lymphoid tissue suggests a role for the appendix in defence against pathogens (see Book 3, Chapter 4), it is clearly not essential as it is commonly removed when inflamed, with no apparent ill-effect.

Summary of Section 4.3.7

1   Most of the water and salts that reach the large intestine are absorbed there.

2   The large intestine is populated by gut bacteria that synthesize vitamin B_{12}, vitamin K, thiamin and riboflavin.

3   Mass movement occurs in the large intestine, often triggered by the entry of food into the stomach.

4   Faeces consist of two-thirds water and one-third solid, including dead bacteria, fibre, small amounts of bile pigments, cholesterol, fatty acids and mucus.

4.4 Disorders of the gut

The absorption of water and mineral salts is of crucial importance to health; normally about 99% of the water and ions that enter the lumen is absorbed. An increase in the amount of water in the faeces is called **diarrhoea**. Diarrhoea can result from disturbance to the processes of both absorption and secretion and causes loss of water and mineral salts from the body. In extreme cases this dehydration can be rapid and fatal although treatment with water and mineral salts is relatively simple. Diarrhoea is usually associated with an increase in gut motility. This also speeds up elimination of the harmful agent. Evidence suggests that both increased secretion and increased motility during diarrhoea can occur by activation of the enteric neurons that control both these processes.

Food poisoning is a common cause of diarrhoea, usually as a result of an infection by food-borne pathogenic microbes such as *Salmonella typhimurium* (*S. typhimurium*), *Escherichia coli* (*E. coli*) and *Staphylococcus aureus* (*S. aureus*) in the intestines. These organisms may release substances that affect ion transport or, in some cases, damage the mucosa. For example, *S. aureus* causes acute gastroenteritis (inflammation of the stomach and intestinal membrane) by the toxins it produces in the food before it is ingested. *S. typhimurium* may be present in meat and poultry, eggs and milk and can cause infection if these products are not cooked thoroughly. *E. coli* can be found in undercooked meat and underpasteurized milk and can cause fatalities in older people.

Coeliac disease is an inflammatory disease of the upper small intestine and results from ingestion of gluten (a protein found in wheat, rye triticale (a hybrid of wheat and rye) and barley) in genetically susceptible individuals. Case Report 4.1 provides a more in-depth look at this relatively common disorder. Coeliac disease can be described as a 'food allergy' as there is evidence of an abnormal immunological reaction to a specific food type. However, the term 'food allergy' is being increasingly used to describe a range of different 'food sensitivities'. Food sensitivities are reproducible unpleasant reactions to a specific food or ingredient which one person gets but others do not get. Food sensitivities can include food aversions with psychological and psychosomatic reactions and food intolerance possibly due to lack of a specific enzyme or irritation.

Inflammatory bowel disease (IBD) is inflammation of the intestine (bowel). Two relatively common IBD conditions are **Crohn's disease** and ulcerative colitis; these conditions are difficult to distinguish between. Both diseases affect young adults (20–40 years) but Crohn's disease causes inflammation deeper into the tissues of the intestinal wall. Crohn's disease affects about 1 in 1000 people in the UK and ulcerative colitis affects about 1 in 600 people in the UK. Both conditions exhibit 'flare-ups' or 'bouts' of pain (which are termed 'exacerbations') and diarrhoea interspersed with periods of remission. Both diseases are treated in a similar manner, with drugs to try and reduce the inflammation and immune system suppressants to maintain remission. Case Report 4.2 on Crohn's disease contains more detail of treatments. In some severe cases surgical removal of the infected part of the bowel is necessary. In these cases an *ileostomy* or *colostomy* is performed in which a piece of the patient's intestine is led from either the ileum or the colon to the outside of the body to allow discharge from the bowel. Sometimes an artificial pipe is used instead.

Colon cancer is the third most frequent cancer after breast and lung cancer. The most important contributing factor is thought to be diet, as populations eating a low-fat high-fibre diet have a very low incidence of this type of cancer. Symptoms of colon cancer include: blood in or on the stools, a change in bowel habit lasting more than six weeks, unexplained weight loss, pain in the abdomen or rectum and a feeling of not having emptied the bowel properly after defaecation. Treatment for bowel cancer will depend on the location and stage of growth of the tumour (if caught early enough the prognosis is good) and may include surgery to remove the tumour and chemotherapy to prevent recurrence of the tumour. Radiotherapy is only used to treat cancer of the rectum and may be offered to support surgery or chemotherapy or both.

Case Report 4.1 Coeliac disease

Janet is a 42-year-old schoolteacher who has found it increasingly difficult to cope with her class of 5- and 6-year-olds. Janet has always enjoyed her job, in which she has worked for the last 20 years. However, lately she has found that she was feeling tired all the time. Janet saw her GP who performed blood tests and these indicated she had mild anaemia. Janet was prescribed iron tablets to resolve the anaemia, but far from feeling better Janet felt even more tired and decided to return to her GP. Her GP took further blood tests, this time looking for a specific type of antibody in the blood called 'IgA anti-endomysium antibody'. The presence of this antibody in the blood indicates that the condition of coeliac disease may be present. The GP also explained to Janet that she may need to have a biopsy (removal of a piece of tissue for diagnostic examination) of her jejunum to confirm a diagnosis of coeliac disease. In coeliac disease the biopsy shows flattening of the villi, which reduces the gut surface area for nutrient absorption.

Janet wanted to know more about the possible implications of coeliac disease and her GP explained that it is an inflammatory disease of the upper small intestine that results, in genetically susceptible individuals, from ingestion of gluten. Inflammation can affect absorption of important nutrients such as iron, folic acid, calcium and fat-soluble vitamins. Many people with coeliac disease have minimal symptoms, that do not seem to be associated with the gut, and simply complain of tiredness like Janet. She was pleased to note that complete remission occurs as a result of permanent withdrawal of gluten from the diet. Recent studies have shown that coeliac disease may affect up to 1 in 200 of the general population.

Gluten should be excluded from the diet of those with coeliac disease. Most of the foods to be avoided will be in the carbohydrate food group and oats may be contaminated so are sometimes also avoided. Baked products such as bread, cakes and biscuits and pizzas all contain gluten and must be avoided, as well as pasta, semolina, breaded products, communion wafer (gluten-free ones are available), thickened products such as pie fillings and some puddings and sauces.

Gluten-free alternatives are available, many on prescription. However, there are a variety of starchy foods that are naturally free from gluten, including rice, rice flour, rice noodles, maize, corn flour, lentils, potatoes, soya beans and soya flour. Other foods that are acceptable and necessary for a healthy balanced diet include all fruits and vegetables, meat, fish, poultry, eggs, nuts, pulses, cheese, milk, yoghurt, oils and spreading fats, tea, coffee and juices. Janet was told that if a diagnosis was confirmed she would be put in touch with a registered dietician who could help her establish a healthy diet and point out some of the possible pitfalls and ways to avoid them.

Case Report 4.2 Crohn's disease

Patricia was 29 years old when she was diagnosed as having Crohn's disease. Although it was an unpleasant shock it was mixed with relief. At last there was a label that could be pinned on her condition to explain why she felt as she did. At the time she was diagnosed Patricia was living alone. Her partner David had moved out of their flat a year earlier and Patricia decided to stay with her sister while she tried to come to terms with her diagnosis.

Patricia had felt unwell on and off for almost two years. At first she had generally felt lethargic and unwell, but over the last year she had increasingly had bouts of diarrhoea, abdominal pain and rectal bleeding and she now found that she was underweight. Patricia became frightened and felt increasingly isolated. When the bouts of diarrhoea occurred, they had become so bad that she began to eat less because she feared not being able to get to a toilet in time to prevent an accident. In fact she felt nervous when going out of the house and had memorized all the functioning toilets on her normal routes. She had begun to carry clean underwear in her handbag, living in fear that an accident would occur, either at work or on her way to or from work. Increasingly, when a bout occurred, Patricia had found the only place she went outside her home was work. She was aware that she was not eating well and that what she was eating did not represent a balanced diet, giving her concern that she was making her general condition worse.

When Patricia was diagnosed she was informed that Crohn's disease is a chronic inflammatory condition that can affect any part of the gastrointestinal tract from the mouth to the anus. However, the mouth, oesophagus and stomach are not usually affected. The most commonly affected parts of the bowel are the ileocaecal region and the colon. The condition can involve several segments of the intestine simultaneously and these regions are commonly referred to as 'skip lesions', the intestine between these areas appearing normal. Crohn's disease is characterized by acute episodes or flare-ups followed by periods of remission, during which people often feel well. Patricia was told the condition is common in western developed countries and tends to affect young people between 20 and 40 years. The cause of Crohn's disease is not known, but it is thought to involve an interaction between genetic factors and environmental agents such as diet, infective agents, smoking and stress.

Patricia was diagnosed through a combination of examinations of stool, laboratory blood investigations, endoscopy (examination of the gut with an endoscope; Figure 4.18), radiological assessment (barium enema) and examination of the cells taken in the biopsy from her rectum, colon and ileum. Patricia was told that Crohn's disease is managed medically in the first instance. Surgery may become necessary due to the complications of the disease such as obstruction of the bowel and development of an intestinal fistulae (an abnormal tract from the lumen of the bowel to the exterior).

Drugs commonly used in Crohn's disease include corticosteroids (anti-inflammatory drugs) and Patricia

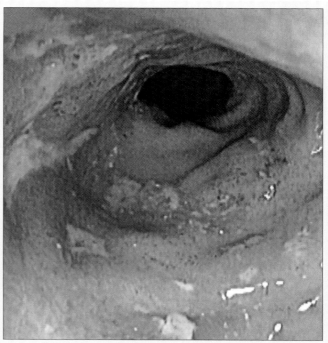

Figure 4.18 Endoscope view of ulceration and inflammation in the ileum.

was started on a course of prednisolone to reduce the inflammation. Patricia was informed that there may be side-effects, although these would be unlikely with low doses of the steroid. Side-effects include increase in weight, increased hair growth, acne, mood changes, high blood pressure and bruising, and prolonged treatment can lead to osteoporosis (reduction in bone density). Importantly, steroids suppress all inflammatory processes and also the generalized reactions of inflammation. This suppression can be very dangerous because the body's method of dealing with infection is impaired and bacteria can spread widely without the seriousness being recognized by either health care professionals or the patient.

Patricia was also informed that other drugs she may need to take include sulfasalazine which can reduce the frequency of exacerbation of the disease. Metronidazole is an antibiotic given to treat infections associated with Crohn's disease and azathioprine can also be given to reduce inflammation.

Patricia was pleased to stay with her sister when newly diagnosed. There was much to consider and much to try to understand.

Summary of Section 4.4

1 Diarrhoea results in loss of water and mineral salts from the body and can lead to severe dehydration and even death.

2 Food poisoning is a common cause of diarrhoea.

3 Coeliac disease is an inflammatory disease of the upper small intestine, caused by ingestion of gluten, a protein found in wheat and other grains.

4 Inflammatory bowel disease (IBD) can be classified into Crohn's disease and ulcerative colitis.

5 Colon cancer is the third most prevalent cancer in the UK; its occurrence is associated with a diet low in fibre and high in fat.

Questions for Chapter 4

Question 4.1 (LOs 4.1–4.4)

Name each of the gut regions and digestive organs labelled A–I in Figure 4.19 and summarize, in the form of a table, the roles of each region, including the activities of the digestive secretions produced.

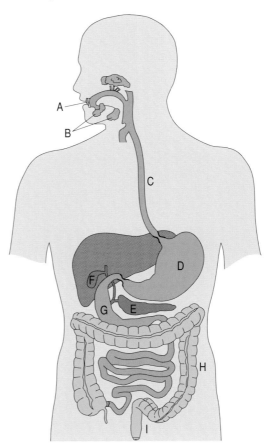

Figure 4.19 For use with Question 4.1.

Question 4.2 (LO 4.2)

Name and briefly describe the two structural specializations of the intestinal epithelium that facilitate absorption of nutrients.

Question 4.3 (LOs 4.2 and 4.3)

Outline what happens to carbohydrates as you eat a meal and they pass along the gut.

Question 4.4 (LOs 4.2 and 4.3)

Outline what happens to proteins as you eat a meal and they pass along the gut.

Question 4.5 (LO 4.4)

Explain how and where amino acids and simple carbohydrates are absorbed in the gut.

Question 4.6 (LOs 4.2 and 4.3)

Explain how fats are digested and absorbed into the body.

Question 4.7 (LO 4.1)

Summarize in a list of bullet points the main roles of the liver.

Question 4.8 (LO 4.5)

Briefly describe the location, symptoms and causes of the following conditions of the digestive tract: (a) gastritis; (b) peptic ulcers; (c) inflammatory bowel disease (IBD); (d) colon cancer.

CONCLUSION

Most of us will have experienced the misery of diarrhoea at some point in our lives. The case report on Crohn's disease must surely leave every one of us who reads it, and who has not had first-hand experience of the disease, nevertheless able to empathize strongly with Patricia's situation. Here we have an account that clearly demonstrates how scientific medicine is able to describe the condition and prescribe treatment to alleviate the symptoms, but is not able to offer an explanation that might allow Patricia to take steps to make a full recovery from the disease. Re-reading the account we notice the implication that relationships have been very important for her. First, in a negative way: the lack of support from a partner, who left a year after she started to feel ill, and her reported feeling of isolation. (Contrast this with the support Mary received from her husband when breast cancer was diagnosed and the encouragement that Ron's wife gave that prompted him to go to his GP.) Subsequently note how pleased Patricia was to stay with her sister when she was newly diagnosed. The support of others at stressful times is obviously of benefit.

We will be describing some of the effects of stress as we continue with the course but already you have probably noted that there are chemicals that are released in stressful situations. The hormones adrenalin and noradrenalin tend to have immediate metabolic effects while the corticosteroids (e.g. cortisol) usually have less immediate but more prolonged effects. The metabolic processes that are influenced by these hormones include increased rates of use of carbohydrates, lipids and proteins. These responses must be interacting with the myriad of processes that are set in train by the ingestion of food and presumably they have a beneficial effect, making energy available to meet the stressful situation effectively. We also read that a corticosteroid is to be given to Patricia, as it has anti-inflammatory properties.

On the other hand we are told that the GP suggests that Crohn's disease may, itself, be brought on by stress. We read in Chapter 1 in connection with wound healing that stress increases vulnerability to disease. We will find out more about stress responses in Book 4 but the indications here are that effects of stress hormones must change over time. When the effects of a metabolite change over time it is quite tricky to prescribe or give advice with confidence.

It is not just changes over time that we have to contend with. Even our short study of digestion has shown that metabolic processes are exceedingly complex. So we have encountered a number of nutrients that are essential in small amounts but deleterious at higher dosages. Examples here are Vitamin A and iron. Whilst attempts are made to give guidance on the recommended and safe levels of intake of nutrients there are difficulties because we are all so tremendously variable in both our genetic make-up and in our lifestyles.

The variability in our ability to metabolize alcohol was seen to have a genetic basis. We may not know which alleles we have inherited but here is an example where we can certainly gauge their effect. This is true for many other reactions. We do get to know our own bodies and how they respond to the way we treat them. It is of no use to someone with lactose intolerance to learn that humans can digest milk and to keep drinking milk. They are not able to digest lactose and drinking milk makes them ill. As the course progresses there will be many examples of variability and divergence from the norm. These may raise questions for you as to what 'normal' is. A more useful consideration may be, in biological terms, to consider always what is 'normal' for any one individual when assessing the condition of good health.

ANSWERS TO QUESTIONS

Question 1.1

The main strength of reductionist approaches to research is that they allow investigations to proceed with great attention to detail on a narrow, and hence manageable front. The intensity of focus on well-defined areas of study has produced the vast wealth of scientific knowledge of the human body and human psychology that informs us today. The weaknesses are twofold. First, the attention to details can be at the expense of attempts to study the whole; influences on a complex phenomenon that fall within the field of study of another discipline are ignored and interactions between different influences go unnoticed. Second, contributions from other fields of study may actually be discredited (for example, some influential biologists have represented sociology as an inferior discipline) thereby damaging competitors for research funding and students.

The main strength of holistic approaches to research is that they seek to understand all the interacting influences on a complex phenomenon. Knowledge generated by one discipline may inform and enhance the investigations carried out in another field of study, and reveal the interactions between them. The weaknesses are that inter-disciplinary studies are intrinsically difficult and complex enterprises; they may not get very far and can produce superficial accounts because so few researchers are fluent in the concepts and methods of more than one discipline. An additional problem is that popularity of holism as a philosophy may be elevating it to the status of a dogma that cannot be criticized – in effect, it may have become the 'new reductionism'!

Question 1.2

The twins should show identical features of growth and development, despite their different environments, since, to a biological determinist, every aspect of their biology is determined by their identical genes.

Question 1.3

The pads of fat are an adaptive characteristic in the Arctic environment, which confers a survival advantage on those individuals who have them. Evolution proceeds by natural selection in which individuals with the most adaptive characteristics in a given environment are 'selected'. These individuals have greater fitness than others, which means they have a greater chance of surviving long enough to reproduce and raise a larger number of offspring relative to others who do not have the fat pads. They pass on their genes to their offspring, who in turn survive to reproduce because they too have the survival advantage conferred by the fat pads. Over many generations, the number of individuals in the population who have the fat pads increases, until everyone has them.

Question 1.4

It is correct to say that epidemiology cannot identify specific causes of conditions such as cardiovascular disease. However, by demonstrating statistically significant correlations, as between hypertension and placental to birth weight ratio in a group of individuals, such studies can lead to the formulation of hypotheses about specific causes of disease which can then be studied by more direct means, leading to ways of improving health.

Question 1.5

You could confirm that heavy smoking does tend to reduce the baby's birth weight, but that it does so by reducing the amount of oxygen and nutrients that the baby receives from the mother. You could point out that this could have long-term consequences for the person's future health, as suggested by epidemiological studies. You might then explain how this could happen through the effects on the blood vessels of the body: reduced oxygen and nutrients for the fetus result in preferential blood flow to the brain, so the body experiences reduced blood pressure and the vessels may then fail to develop normal elasticity, which could be irreversible. Finally, to reassure her, you could add that there are many built-in protective factors for the fetus, and that reasonable care is all that is required for a successful childbirth.

Question 2.1

The three-dimensional shape of haemoglobin is determined by its primary structure (i.e. by the sequence of amino acids in the chains). When the chains fold to form the 3-D shape the negative charge on glutamic acid will help to stabilize the shape by forming a bond, a bond that cannot be formed when the non-polar valine replaces it in position 6.

The abnormal haemoglobin causes the red blood cells to become sickle shaped, instead of having the normal disc shape.

Question 2.2

The enzyme forms part of the system that controls ATP production. When levels of ATP rise some will bind to the enzyme and thereby reduce the enzyme's activity. When ATP levels drop, ATP molecules detach from the enzyme and the enzyme becomes active again. This is an example of negative feedback and it ensures that the level of ATP, the cell's energy currency, can be matched to requirements.

Question 2.3

(a) Mitochondria are the 'powerhouses' of the cell and new-born babies can therefore generate a lot of heat by the 'fat-burning' activity of the numerous mitochondria. (In fact, brown fat mitochondria are specially adapted to producing heat in preference to generating energy as ATP.)

(b) The Golgi sacs process (in this instance, add sugar chains to) the proteins destined for export as mucus. The proteins are synthesized by ribosomes on the ER. Vesicles containing the finished product (the mucus glycoprotein) bud off from the Golgi sacs and move up the cell to fuse with the cell membrane and so release their contents into the lumen of the intestine.

Question 2.4

A portion of DNA receives a signal that causes it to unwind and separate into two strands. RNA is made using the template strand. This is transcription. mRNA leaves the nucleus and enters the cytosol. Here ribosomes attach to it. The mRNA/ribosome complex is the site of keratin synthesis, the process being known as translation. The mRNA has a finite life so keratin will only be manufactured for as long as the template DNA is exposed and is being transcribed.

Question 2.5

After a cell has duplicated all its cellular components, including its DNA, the nuclear membrane disappears and the chromosomes gather at the centre of the cell. A mitotic apparatus forms with two poles from which fibres radiate and attach to one of each pair of duplicated chromosomes. One of each type of chromosome then moves, pulled by the contracting fibres, to each pole and a new nuclear membrane forms around each complete set of chromosomes. Finally, the cytoplasm between the nuclei contracts, resulting in the separation into two identical daughter cells.

Question 2.6

Persistent tenderness and redness of the skin indicates that the inflammation and early repair phases are being prolonged. Blood vessels are enlarged, releasing cells that clear up debris at the site of damage, and fibroblasts lay down new connective tissue. A cause of the delay in healing is likely to be the stress experienced by the carer, which reduces such factors as the level of interleukin in white cells, resulting in decreased fibroblast activity and slower connective tissue formation.

You might advise your friend to:

*   arrange some relief from the care-giving until the wound heals properly;

*   eat a healthier diet so that nutrition is optimal;

*   seek medical assistance.

Question 3.1

Fibre helps to bulk up the food as it passes through the gut, helping to prevent diverticular disease and minimizing transit times and contact time between any toxic substances in the food (which might trigger cancer) and the cells of the gut. Diets high in fibre are usually low in fat and non-milk extrinsic sugars and high in micronutrients, thus helping to produce a balanced, healthy diet.

Question 3.2

Human diseases and disorders are rarely caused by one single factor – diet is usually only one of many contributing factors. It is difficult to isolate any effect a dietary component may have from these other factors. Food is usually made from a complex mixture of different substances and it may be the interaction between these components, rather than an individual component, that is important.

Question 3.3

(a) The body mass index (BMI) of an individual can be calculated to determine whether they are within the healthy range for their height:

$$\text{BMI} = \frac{\text{weight/kg}}{(\text{height/m})^2}$$

(b) Sarah: $\text{BMI} = \dfrac{55}{1.65^2} = \dfrac{55}{2.7225} = 20.2$

Ian: $\text{BMI} = \dfrac{88}{1.84^2} = \dfrac{88}{3.3856} = 25.99 = 26$

Sarah is classified as within the healthy weight range, although she needs to take care not to lose any weight as she is at the bottom of the range.

Ian is classified as overweight and should be advised to try and lose weight. Ian should be encouraged to lose weight now as he is only just in the overweight classification and it would be sensible to lose the small amount of weight necessary to put him in the healthy weight range.

(c) Having calculated your own BMI reflect on whether this affects your perception of your body image. If your BMI falls outside of the 'desirable' range it would be sensible to consult your GP for advice even if you think you are 'just fine'.

Question 3.4

Sodium, potassium and calcium ions all have a vital role in communication by neurons.

Other minerals are important for communication in the endocrine system, as they form an essential component of some hormones (e.g. iodine is an essential component of thyroid hormones).

Vitamins are also important for communication in the body. Vitamin A and D derivatives act as signalling molecules inside cells, affecting gene transcription and hence the properties of cells. For example, vitamin D promotes transcription of the gene encoding the calcium-binding protein on the surface of interstitial epithelial cells, and hence promotes absorption of calcium from the gut.

Question 3.5

The child is normally boisterous so probably usually eats a healthy balanced diet: suppression of appetite when unwell is common. Lying in bed uses less energy than usual (although extra energy is needed for repair and recovery) but sugar provides a good supply of energy and the child's TEI is probably adequate. It might be worth trying to stimulate the appetite with something like peanuts (Table 3.9), a high-protein snack enjoyed by most youngsters, as protein requirements are higher during periods of recovery. Vitamin usage can also be higher when fighting infection so consideration should be given to a vitamin supplement. Of course the parents should consult their GP if recovery is slow or if they have any other concerns.

Question 4.1

Table 4.4 summarizes the digestive activities of structures A–I in Figure 4.19.

Question 4.2

The epithelium has many finger-like projections, called villi, and the absorptive cell membrane of individual epithelial cells has many small projections, called microvilli, which form the brush border. These specializations greatly increase the surface area through which absorption can take place.

Question 4.3

Digestion of carbohydrates begins in the mouth, where they are mixed with amylase produced by the salivary glands. This enzyme breaks down starch into polysaccharide chains of shorter lengths. Soon after food reaches the stomach, the salivary amylase is denatured by hydrochloric acid (HCl). The HCl also assists in carbohydrate digestion by releasing carbohydrates from bulky foods. When the food reaches the small intestine, pancreatic amylase continues the digestion of the polysaccharide chains into disaccharides and short chains of glucose (called dextrins). The digestion of these into monosaccharides is completed by enzymes situated on the brush border of the intestinal epithelium. The monosaccharides are then absorbed by Na$^+$-coupled active transport. Non-digestible plant polysaccharides (fibre) pass to the large intestine, where some are digested by harmless bacteria, producing gases. The bulky undigested plant polysaccharides are important for the formation and movement of faeces, and are also linked to reduced occurrence of colon cancer, heart disease and diabetes.

Table 4.4 Answer to Question 4.1.

Gut region or digestive organ	Digestive secretion	Functions
A mouth (jaw, teeth and tongue)		chewing, initiation of swallowing reflexes
B salivary glands	mineral salts and water	moistens food
	mucus	lubricates food
	amylase	begins breakdown of polysaccharides
C oesophagus		moves food to stomach by peristalsis
D stomach	hydrochloric acid (HCl) mucus pepsin (from pepsinogen)	stores, mixes, dissolves and begins main digestion of food; regulates passage of partially digested food (chyme) into small intestine
		dissolves food; activates pepsinogen; kills microbes
		lubricates and protects epithelial surface
		begins protein digestion
E pancreas	bicarbonate (HCO$_3^-$)	neutralizes HCl entering small intestine from stomach
	proteolytic enzymes, amylase, lipase and nucleases	digest proteins, polysaccharides, lipids and nucleic acids, respectively
F gall bladder		stores bile between meals and releases it into small intestine as required
G small intestine	disaccharide-splitting and proteolytic enzymes which are not secreted but are present in brush borders of epithelial cells	mixing and propulsion of contents by peristalsis
	enzyme (enterokinase) that activates a pancreatic proteolytic enzyme (trypsin)	complete digestion of carbohydrates and proteins absorption of products of digestion
H colon	mucus	storage and digestion of non-digestible matter; mixing and propulsion of contents by peristalsis
		lubrication of faeces
I rectum		defaecation

Question 4.4

Protein digestion starts in the stomach where the hydrochloric acid (HCl) denatures proteins making a larger surface area for proteases to act upon. Pepsin starts the proteolytic digestion of ingested proteins in the stomach and the pancreatic enzymes trypsin, chymotrypsin, elastase and carboxypeptidase continue this process. Aminopeptidase in the brush border of the small intestine is also involved in breaking peptides into individual amino acids. Amino acids are actively transported from the lumen of the gut into the epithelial cells.

Question 4.5

Amino acid absorption occurs in the small intestine by active transport using specific transporter proteins in the apical membrane of the epithelial cell. Sodium ions (Na$^+$) are cotransported with the amino acids and ATP is used to fuel the process. The amino acids leave the epithelial cell by a number of processes to enter the blood capillary on the basal side of the cell.

Monosaccharides (e.g. glucose, galactose and fructose) are also absorbed in the small intestine. A family of glucose transporter proteins transports glucose and galactose into the epithelial cells. Sodium ions are cotransported at the same time and the transport is active as the monosaccharides are pumped across the membrane. Fructose apparently crosses the membrane into the cell by facilitated diffusion. The monosaccharides leave the epithelial cell by facilitated diffusion and enter the capillaries.

Question 4.6

Fats need to be emulsified before efficient enzymic digestion can occur. This emulsification is facilitated by bile salts and it increases the surface area of the fat to the action of lipase. Lipase digests triacylglycerols into monoacylglycerol molecules and two fatty acids. These breakdown products (along with bile salts and phospholipids) form micelles that act as a reservoir of monoacylglycerol and fatty acid molecules. These molecules can simply diffuse down their concentration gradient across the apical membrane of the epithelial cell and into the cell where they then reform triacylglycerol molecules. This (along with sequestration into chylomicrons in the endoplasmic reticulum) ensures that the concentration of free fatty acids inside the cell is kept low hence maintaining the concentration difference across the apical membrane of the cell. The chylomicrons are released from the Golgi in vesicles that fuse with the basal cell membrane and release them into the interstitial fluid between cells. The chylomicrons cannot pass through the capillary walls and so enter the lymph vessels and then are transported to the bloodstream.

Question 4.7

The liver has a number of roles:

* digestion by the formation of bile which aids in fat emulsification and release of bicarbonate ions which help neutralize the acidic chyme on leaving the stomach;

* maintenance of blood glucose levels;

* metabolism of fats including cholesterol and triacylglycerols;

- metabolism of proteins including synthesis of blood plasma proteins and urea production from amino acid breakdown;

- excretion and detoxification of noxious substances and destruction of old red blood cells, producing bile;

- storage of fat-soluble vitamins and iron and copper;

- heat production.

Question 4.8

(a) *Gastritis* occurs in the stomach when there is too much gastric juice and too little mucus to protect the stomach mucosa from the acidity. Symptoms of gastritis are stomach cramps, pain and nausea. There are various causes of gastritis including excessive alcohol consumption, food poisoning, heavy smoking and prolonged use of aspirin.

(b) *Peptic ulcers* occur in the stomach when the mucosa is eroded. Symptoms of ulcers often occur on ingestion of food and include nausea, heartburn, discomfort and pain. The causes of peptic ulcers are unclear but a bacterial infection of *Helicobacter pylori* is often found in patients.

(c) *Inflammatory bowel disease* (*IBD*) can occur anywhere in the digestive tract and is chronic inflammation of the intestine. IBD can be classified into Crohn's disease and ulcerative colitis and both these conditions exhibit bouts of pain and diarrhoea.

(d) *Colon cancer* is cancer of the colon. Symptoms include blood in or on the stools, a change of bowel habit that lasts more than six weeks, unexplained weight loss, pain in the stomach or rectum and a feeling of not having emptied the bowel properly after defaecation. One of the contributing factors to colon cancer is thought to be a low-fibre and high-fat diet.

ACKNOWLEDGEMENTS

Grateful acknowledgement is made to the following sources for permission to reproduce material within this product.

Figures

Figure 1.2: Larsen, W. J. (1993) *Human Embryology*, Churchill Livingstone; *Figure 1.3*: Gilbert, S. G. (1989) *Pictorial Human Embryology*, University of Washington Press; *Figure 1.4a*: Copyright © Alamy Images; *Figure 1.4b*: Mike Levers. Copyright © The Open University; *Figures 1.5a and 1.7b*: Science Photo Library; *Figure 1.5b*: Laguan Design/Science Photo Library; *Figure 1.7a*: Courtesy of Paul Gabbott/Open University; *Figure 1.8*: Biophoto Asssociates/Science Photo Library; *Figure 1.11*: Strickberger, M. W. (1985) *Genetics*, Blackie and Son Ltd; *Figure 1.13a and b*: Adapted from Smith, C. P. W. and Williams, P. L. (1984) *Basic Human Embryology*, 3rd edn, Churchill Livingstone.

Figure 2.1: Science Photo Library; *Figure 2.12*: Biophoto Associates/Science Photo Library; *Figure 2.13b*: Perry, M. M. and Gilbert, A. B. (1979) *Journal of Cell Science*, **39**, p. 266, The Company of Biologists Ltd; *Figure 2.18a, b*: Courtesy of Mike Stewart/Open University; *Figure 2.18c*: Ed Reschke; *Figure 2.18d*: Courtesy of Caroline Pond/Open University; *Figure 2.23*: Copyright © Dorothy F. Bainton; *Figure 2.24*: Kiecolt-Glaser, J. K., Marucha, P. T., Malarkey, W. B., Mercado, A. M. and Glaser, R. (1995) 'Slowing of wound healing by psychological stress', *The Lancet*, **346**, p. 1195, November 1995, Lancet Ltd.

Figure 3.1: British Nutrition Foundation, www.nutrition.org.uk concept for the Balance of Good Health Model, copyright Food Standards Agency; *Figure 3.3*: Alberts, B., Bray, D., Lewis, J., Raff, M. Roberts, K. and Watson, J. D. (1994) *Molecular Biology of the Cell*, Garland Publishing Inc.; *Figure 3.4*: Mauro Fermariello/Science Photo Library; *Figure 3.5*: Bender, D. A. (1993) *An Introduction to Nutrition and Metabolism*, Taylor and Francis; *Figure 3.11*: Waugh, A. and Grant, A. (2001) *Anatomy and Physiology in Health and Illness*, Churchill Livingstone.

Figures 4.5, 4.7, 4.8 and 4.9: Reprinted from Waugh, A. and Grant A. (2001) *Anatomy and Physiology in Health and Illness*, 9th edn, pp. 289, 291, 290, 295, with permission from Elsevier; *Figures 4.11 (inset) and 4.18*: Science Photo Library; *Figures 4.12, 4.13, 4.15 and 4.17*: Vander, A. J., Sherman, J. H. and Luciano, D. S. (2001) *Human Physiology, The Mechanisms of Body Function*, 8th international edition, copyright © 2001, 1998, 1994, 1990, 1985, 1980, 1975, 1970 by McGraw-Hill, Inc., with permission of The McGraw-Hill Companies; *Figure 4.14*: Alberts, B. et al. (2002) *Molecular Biology of the Cell*, Routledge/Taylor & Francis Books, Inc.

Tables

Table 1.1: Barker, D. J. P. (1992) 'Foetal and infant origins of adult disease', *British Medical Journal*, **304** (6820), p. 178, January 1992, BMJ Publishing.

Every effort has been made to contact copyright holders. If any have been inadvertently overlooked the publishers will be pleased to make the necessary arrangements at the first opportunity.

INDEX

Entries and page numbers in **bold type** refer to key words which are printed in **bold** in the text. Page numbers in italics are for items mainly or wholly in a figure or table.